CW00969537

HOW T
A CANCER
PATIENT

HOW TO BE A CANCER PATIENT

A Proven Approach for Optimizing Your Role in Your Cancer Treatment

JEFF BOOTHMAN

Published by Igniting Souls Publishing Agency
Powell, Ohio
www.ignitingsouls.com

Identifiers:
LCCN:2022921813
ISBN: 979-8-88583-161-1 (paperback)
ISBN: 979-8-88583-162-8 (hardback)
ISBN: 979-8-88583-164-2 (ebook)

Available in paperback, hardback, e-book, and audiobook.

NOTE TO EVERY CANCER PATIENT

Here is one of the things no one really tells you about having cancer. I believe it is important, so I have it out front.

More people than you ever will know are pulling for you. I am five years out as I finish writing this, and I still, to this day, see people I haven't seen since my diagnosis who told me they were praying for me. They were acquaintances or friends of friends I never knew very well or even at all in some cases.

When you feel down, realize that who and what you see supporting you is really only the tip of the iceberg. The support for you is much deeper than you will ever realize. The support, prayers, and good feelings sent on your behalf are a welcoming foundation upon which you can rest when you have tough days. When you are alone, scared, or tired, reflect on this simple fact and let it fill you with strength and determination.

I will pray for you and wish you the best. Please know that even when you feel most alone, there are probably thousands of people all over the world, most you have never met, with their hands on your back.

Whether you think you can or you think you can't— you're right.

—Henry Ford

CONTENTS

FOREWORD

There is a koan in Zen Buddhism that states, "Make medicine from suffering." The intent of this koan is to ask us to look at how we view tragedy in life and then what we do with those experiences. The goal is to see what we can do with what life brings us—not only for our own lives but for the best interests of others. When we can see that we are all patients in the same hospital seeking to get well, we may recognize that we may or may not be taking the medicine "life" is prescribing and can seek to become our own doctors. We may then become a doctor for others to help them see their way to healing, and collectively, we can become part of the solution for what ails us all. It is likely that every one of us has or will have a connection to someone diagnosed with cancer. Given this fact, it may behoove us all to heed these wise words sown by a wise Buddhist master—whether we are the patient, family member, friend, or physician—to see how we can find healing physically, emotionally, or spiritually, for ourselves and others. I firmly believe this book is part of the solution to do precisely that.

The incidence of cancers in type and diagnoses is on the rise, as many of us may seem to hear in our circles of friends, family, and media. Research indicates there could be a 49% rise in the number of diagnoses in the next few decades, mostly because we are living longer, as well as other issues and concerns that could drive those statistics. While cancer rates may be increasing, early detection and advances in treatment are decreasing the mortality rate. With this in mind, we should be of the mind that what seemed to feel like a grim diagnosis at one time is now possibly seen as simply another rock or boulder on our journey. In my field of psychology, while attitude is not everything, it definitely is a major contributor to outcomes. Therefore, the many factors that may affect our attitudes are significant issues that may affect our cancer outcomes and our short- and long-term recovery. I believe our feelings, emotions, and beliefs about the treatment process and our empowerment in that process are significant. Factors that can help to improve our attitude toward our cancer and treatment are so important, and most importantly, our sense of awareness of what we may expect while going through the process can contribute to healthier (or unhealthier) paths through treatment.

While medical professionals treat cancers every day, they are often not very adept at providing a roadmap for the experiences, emotions, and processes involved in the journey. Because of this, for many patients and support people the journey can be fraught with fears, concerns, questions, and doubts. *How to Be a Cancer Patient* does a great job of providing a perspective of the journey through the eyes of a cancer patient. It provides a plethora of tips and insights and is extremely helpful through a chronicling of the experiences that will be helpful, not only for the patient but for all of those involved in the cancer journey.

Jeff has definitely made medicine from suffering and shares his healing journey with all who choose to read this book. Written through the eyes of a problem solver, Jeff looks keenly at the challenges he experienced and likely face many cancer patients and the health-care system that cares for them. I have known Jeff for more than 30 years and have always known him to be, in both his life and work, an incisive problem solver. As the Little Dutch Boy was able to demonstrate the wisdom in sticking his finger in the dike, Jeff has used his skillset to provide sound, simple guidance that others may have overlooked. Being an outside observer of the system and seeing some of the challenges and providing common sense solutions hopefully can ease the journey for many—not only physically but emotionally. While all too often the cancer journey's focus is on medical health, both Jeff and I see the importance of not ignoring the mental health aspects of the journey. As a licensed psychologist for three decades, I believe that mental health practitioners should be a part of every treatment team to assess chronic and situational stress, treatment compliance, and personality dynamics as they may affect treatment and outcome, family, and community support systems, and other factors that may affect treatment and long-term prognosis. For anyone going through this journey (patient or family member) who is feeling difficulty with coping, both Jeff and I ask that you please seek some help from a mental health professional.

We are all in this together.

Erik Fisher, PhD, aka Dr. E.
Licensed Psychologist
www.DrEPresents.com

1

WHY I WROTE THIS BOOK

The purpose of life is to contribute in some way
to make things better.
—Robert F. Kennedy

When I was officially diagnosed with cancer, I pretty much knew it was coming (learn about exactly how a little later in the book); but I didn't know the specifics. When my doctor finally told me, it was very clinical. "We got the results from pathology, and you have T-cell lymphoma."

Next, we discussed the treatment plan, timing, and some of the specifics of what was to come. It was about five o'clock in the evening the day before Thanksgiving. My wife started crying.

Well, that sucks, I thought. They told me I was sick but never told me or taught me how to deal with what was to come. That's where this book comes in.

Cancer is a huge mental and organizational challenge and can feel overwhelming, to say the least. I believe a process and a plan to navigate treatment will assist many, if not all, cancer patients as they walk through their cancer journey so they can do their part to make sure their treatment is as effective as possible and with the least amount of stress for them and those who support them.

This book provides key strategies for managing yourself, your actions, and your mindset as you navigate your cancer journey. It gives the patient and their advocates a plan to manage themselves through their treatment. It is, essentially, coaching to help you manage your role in your cancer treatment.

WHY DON'T HOSPITALS DO THIS?

As I thought about why a hospital doesn't really provide a process and a plan for cancer patients to manage themselves to be super effective as patients, I came up with a few observations:

1. Hospitals manage the processes they use to deliver care. They don't spend a lot of time developing resources to help patients effectively manage themselves through a treatment process. There are available resources, but there generally is no structured approach to guiding patients through the mental and organizational challenges of a long-term treatment process like cancer treatment.

2. Most non-primary mental health challenges (*i.e.*, stresses from cancer treatment) are resolved when patients "opt in" to resources. An example is that when patients seek out additional mental health support when the stress of treatment becomes acute. Now, think of men asking for driving directions (or directions of any sort), and you can start to see the possible disconnect here. *Sometimes you don't even know you need help.*

3. Hospitals don't always encourage patients to challenge their staff to find areas of compromise or process alternatives during patient interactions. When you continually advocate (politely) for yourself, it puts additional pressure on standard care processes. Some hospitals and treatment centers are open to this; some aren't.

4. Hospitals don't get paid to help patients manage themselves through the treatment process of a long-term illness; they get paid to treat the medical problem—in this case, cancer.

I'm no expert on hospitals, but I am an expert in being able to deconstruct any type of operation to understand exactly how they function, so I'd guess that these observations I've made are pretty close to the mark.

I 100% believe that every hospital does everything they can to help patients get better. Additionally, I don't think they are set up to deliver and implement a structured process and plan to coach everyone they treat to be as effective as possible as patients. It's much more than simply letting your care team do their jobs; it's a participation sport if you are a patient.

It's a Big Coaching Opportunity

Think about this: we give five-year-old kids more coaching before their first soccer game than we do cancer patients fighting for their lives. It's ridiculous.

I am convinced the lack of a process to manage the mental challenge of cancer diagnosis and treatment is an enormous opportunity in cancer care and recovery. A good mental and organizational strategy for dealing with the cancer treatment process from diagnosis through recovery can make the difference between success or failure in your treatment—life or death for some people, really.

During my treatment, I spent fifteen days inpatient in the hospital—some scheduled, some not. This included a fine needle aspiration (not a huge procedure but a good story), two surgeries, three rounds of inpatient chemo (at least four days each time), one blood transfusion, some unscheduled days in the hospital, some extra scans due to complications, and then fifteen doses of radiation. After that, I was sent on my way, as good as new but also much smarter about the business of being a cancer patient. I worked, over time, to build myself into the best cancer patient possible.

As I walked the halls of the hematology-oncology floor at the James Cancer Center at The Ohio State University, I saw hundreds of cancer patients during my impatient days. They were in hospital beds, getting treatments, shots, scans, operations, and everything else that could be done to cancer patients. It was pretty much all the awful stuff you see in hospitals on TV, except they were all in one place and not actors.

I witnessed many people I knew who, for sure, would give up and die. You could see it in their eyes. (I'm crying as I write this, and I'm not a big crier.) It feels horrible, and unless you are able to detach, it can affect you—a lot. I told myself that when I got better, I would find a way to help cancer patients somehow. This book is only the beginning.

What I noticed was the people, specifically the patients, and how they were reacting to being cancer patients. I saw every conceivable response: some people were joking around with nervous energy, some were very serious, some were sad, and others were on their way to giving up. There were also a lot of people who were simply overwhelmed. My guess was they really didn't have a place to start to deal with what was happening to them—or at least what was going on in their head. Honestly, I started watching patients in the hospital to try to find a role model or example to follow. It didn't work out too well; it turns out I can't read minds.

I spoke with many doctors, nurses, social workers, patient advocates, chaplains, and medical professionals during my days in the hospital and clinics. They confirmed a lot of what I observed, either directly or indirectly. They kept asking questions as if I was in a totally different headspace than where I actually was. Social workers asked about anxiety. The patient advocates asked about stress and what the medical team could do to comfort me.

The chaplain visits were probably the most interesting, however. The first one who visited asked how I was doing and dealing with my diagnosis and whether I needed spiritual assistance. I told her, in so many words, that I was good. She seemed unconvinced by my words, and we talked for quite a while over a few visits. More on that story later, but her surprise and observations from visits with other patients were a revelation for me. (I know, maybe not the best word to use here.)

HOW I THINK ABOUT STUFF

When I was in graduate school, I took a course in cybernetics. It's a big fancy word, but in a nutshell, it means the study of systems. A system could be an ecosystem, a parking lot filling and emptying, a method of maximizing revenue for an airplane flight—pretty much any group of independent but interrelated entities whose interactions impact how the whole system functions via some type of feedback loop or loops. We learned structured approaches to analyze wildly diverse systems to get a very in-depth understanding of how, exactly, they functioned.

The ability to structure a review of complex systems is probably the best life skill I learned at any level of education. This type of analysis framework defines many of the lenses I use to see the world. It also helped me sort out in unique ways a lot of what I experienced as a patient.

IT'S ABOUT A PROCESS AND A PLAN

I watch a lot of college football. My wife says too much sometimes. That may be true, but I do learn from it at times. One of my favorite examples of having a process is the University of Alabama Football coach, Nick Saban, who is famous for preaching "the process." What does that mean, exactly? It's a series of principles he has his team live by to manage themselves, their efforts, and their experiences in every moment and, most importantly, purposely.

It turns out that *all* cancer patients need something similar—not only those who "opt in" to additional mental health resources. This book provides a process to manage thoughts about being sick and a plan for cancer patients to manage themselves through treatment and beyond.

When you combine systems thinking with recognizing the value of a structured process, you come up with the strategies found in this book.

Here are four realities that make this book immensely useful:

1. You never really know what is going on inside someone's head. With cancer and cancer treatment, there are always very good reasons for patients to be a little incomplete in expressing how they are feeling when talking to family, friends, co-workers, etc. Sometimes it's purposely, while other times, they simply can't express their feelings.

2. People are often reluctant to ask for help, especially when feeling overwhelmed. Sometimes they don't even know what help would be useful. As a patient, you can get a little lost. It can be paralyzing.

3. Most of the readily available help for cancer patients via websites, books, or pamphlets is very general. I have found they are mostly long lists of very general suggestions, leaving the patient to research the best way for them to meditate, deal with doctors, stress, or whatever. The last thing you need when you have cancer is another research assignment. This book offers specific suggestions and starting points for most of the mental and organizational challenges you will encounter. Use the ones that resonate with you.

4. Finally, and most importantly, EVERY cancer patient can benefit from a defined approach to manage their journey and maximize the benefit of their participation in their treatment and recovery. I hope you can view me as a coach with an approach that will help you manage yourself as a cancer patient.

Now let's get to it. Lets start the work of building you into the best cancer patient possible.

Disclaimer: This isn't medical advice. I am not a doctor, but instead, I am an experienced survivor.

2
THE APPROACH

Give me six hours to chop down a tree, and I will spend
the first four sharpening the axe.

—Abraham Lincoln

THE SIX IMPORTANT TOOLS: MANAGED HEAD-
SPACE, ADVOCATING, STUDIED INDIFFERENCE,
TOUGHNESS AND DETERMINATION, DECIDED
FAITH, AND FEARLESSNESS

I don't believe the recipe for success in navigating your treatment is
complicated. In fact, it's pretty simple. You can use the few select
strategies and tools in this book to manage the stresses that come
with a cancer diagnosis and the management of your treatment. I will
touch on each of these tools briefly before diving deeper and providing
you with ways to apply these concepts in each of the individual sections.

The following sections are ordered sequentially based on when you
would likely need them in your progression through treatment.

How to Think: Get Yourself Together"or Managed Headspace

What It Is: Managed Headspace refers to the need to develop skills
in managing your thoughts during cancer treatment while also con-
trolling what you allow to enter into your thought patterns.

Why It Matters: you have the ability to suffer or thrive mentally during your treatments. You can only thrive if you manage your thoughts.

How to Do This: in short, you manage what you think and think about <u>very purposefully</u> until you focus as much as possible on successful treatment and recovery.

How to Advocate: Advocate for Yourself

What It Is: you are advocating for yourself to work <u>with</u> your treatment team to get the best resources and the most flexibility available during your treatment.

Why It Matters: you are at the center of your treatment team, and it is in your best interest to be the information coordinator and process accountant for your treatment.

How to Do This: step up, ask questions, and ask for anything and everything that may make your treatment as effective and comfortable as possible.

How to Act: Studied Indifference

What It Is: a process to become FULLY informed about your treatment and then be able to sit back and let the treatment happen with full knowledge and confidence of exactly what should and could happen— both good and bad.

Why It Matters: it is the least stressful way to pilot yourself through the actual hands-on cancer treatments you will receive.

How to Do This: get very disciplined at using a process to ask questions about your treatment plan (present and near future) to allow for a complete understanding of what is going to occur medically and the possible physical and emotional consequences. This allows you to gather all the information needed to be as comfortable as possible with your treatment <u>before</u> it happens.

<u>How to Think: Toughness Response</u>

What It Is: realizing some pain or difficulty is coming and deciding on purpose, to step up to the challenge and persevere.

Why It Matters: a Toughness Response is essential to help you stay out of the ruts that can grab you when you are experiencing a lot of pain, nausea, or other side effects during treatment.

How to Do This: know the challenge is coming, determine where you will gather strength from, and then act if or when the challenge arrives.

<u>How to Think: Applied Determination</u>

What It Is: deciding (on purpose and ahead of time) to make small steps to (re)gain confidence in resuming your normal life.

Why It Matters: Applied Determination is a crucial step to maintaining some control over what you are planning and doing while allowing you to build momentum in working to resume a normal life.

How to Do This: set your goal, find an accountability partner, and then execute (and celebrate).

<u>How to Think: Decided Faith</u>

What It Is: this is purposeful recognition of the role your faith has in helping you navigate your cancer journey.

Why It Matters: faith helps focus attention and offers support as you work through the challenges of diagnosis and treatment.

How to Do This: understand where you are in your faith journey and use that knowledge to develop leverage based on faith to push through the physically and emotionally difficult times. You must also have faith in yourself <u>and</u> your treatment because it can be difficult to let faith in from other sources if it doesn't start from within.

<u>How to Think: Be Fearless</u>

What It Is: a general approach to stop being worried about your cancer returning and simply deciding to live your life when your treatment is done.

Why It Matters: life after cancer can feel scary for people who fear its return or love the attention that having cancer can bring.

How to Do This: do your part to let your follow-up care team know exactly how you are doing at each checkup, then purposefully decide to leave cancer behind and live fearlessly, courageously, and passionately. As a psychologist friend of mine often asks, "Are you living to die or dying to live?"

3

DIAGNOSIS—"GET YOURSELF TOGETHER" OR MANAGED HEADSPACE

Get yourself together.

—Homer Smith, football coach

I listen to Rick Neuheisel on sports radio. He has a great quote he learned from one of his football coaches along the way. When someone on the team was flustered, not paying attention, or didn't know what to do, this coach would tell the player, "Get yourself together."

My guess is that you felt flustered, detached, or didn't know what to do the exact second you found out you had cancer. You probably needed someone to tell you to "get yourself together", I know I did. Maybe you still need someone to tell you that now.

When your doctor gave you your official diagnosis, you probably felt like there were a million things that all happened at once. You probably had someone close to you when you went for your test results or diagnosis, and it is also likely that you both got emotional. Maybe you received the news over the phone or possibly in the doctor's office. Whatever the case, the doctor likely gave you a ton of information in a very short period of time. You may have started to think about different outcomes. Perhaps you started generating a list of questions while all of this information was swirling in your head.

If you're like me, you likely lost your focus. While you might remember 10% of all of the presented information, you definitely remember 100% of the feelings of fear and worry. (Your personal math may vary some, but I would guess it's pretty close to this.) Regardless of the exact percentages, you started thinking about your prognosis in earnest right after your "official" diagnosis.

After that, you likely started finding things to worry about (or started "officially" worrying about things you already thought about). Just like that, you started moving toward a pretty big and very unproductive rabbit hole. It's a natural reaction.

No matter where you are in your journey, make it a point to begin managing your thoughts and awareness of what you are allowing yourself to focus on. You need to get a handle on your thoughts, emotions, and focus. Say whatever you say to yourself to "get yourself together," but do it—RIGHT NOW. Whining, complaining, and allowing your emotions (fear, worry, freakouts) to overwhelm clear thinking is not helpful. So stop it. If you need help, there are a few strategies listed at the end of this chapter. Go start working the problem.

Get yourself together.

If all of this is too much for you to sort out in your head, raise your hand and ask for professional help or support. There are always resources. Don't wait.

With or without professional help, stick with me. I'll provide you with some tools and methods in this chapter to help you start wrangling your thoughts. It's one of the most important things you can do. It's urgent and important. Quadrant 1 for all you Covey fans. It's the foundational process of the book.

THE GARDEN ANALOGY

I like to garden. I started gardening years ago so I could make homemade salsa with fresh and sometimes unique ingredients (*i.e.*, Black Prince tomatoes). I grow all sorts of stuff now, including tomatoes, onions, garlic, peppers, raspberries, beans, potatoes— you get the picture.

A few years ago, my wife and I moved to a different house with a lot more land. I was very excited because it gave me room for a huge garden and more of everything planted, including some new additions—or so I thought. I cleared the existing (pretty big) garden of weeds, tilled the soil, and then planted a ton of stuff—all the normal salsa garden ingredients, Japanese corn (for popcorn), and some unique melons. We tended the garden every day and watered it whenever Mother Nature was not cooperating.

About mid-summer, we always go on a family vacation for a week. It rained a bunch while we were gone, so we figured we were all set; the plants would have plenty of water and wouldn't be too dry. Hot and wet weather was perfect for the garden. When we got back from vacation, I was pretty excited to see how much things had grown. After all, it was our biggest garden EVER, so I was hoping for great things. I unpacked my suitcase some before I went out for the garden inspection. Immediately, I noticed two issues: there were a ton of weeds growing, and 99% of the green beans were gone, courtesy of the deer or some other animals. No bueno.

I'm pretty sure you aren't reading this book to hear all about my gardening adventures, but I think it's a very fitting analogy for what happens in your head and with your thinking and feeling when you are diagnosed with cancer if you let it. So stick with me.

When your doctor tells you that you have cancer, it opens up a new place in your brain where you store and contemplate thoughts, fears, ideas, and questions about your diagnosis, treatment, survival, etc. I call it the cancer headspace. Exactly what you allow to get into and stay in your cancer headspace can become the foundation, at least in part, of how you respond during your cancer journey.

You may have thought about what your diagnosis could mean to you before you knew for sure that you had cancer. Now that you know for certain you have cancer, it's totally different; it's very real. It can feel scary and overwhelming, but it doesn't have to be.

At the point you are told that you are sick, you have three choices regarding your cancer headspace:

1. You let all your fears and worries occupy this space in your head and keep focusing on those fears and worries over and over. (It's like the weeds in the garden, growing fast.) This is bad, so don't do this.

2. You let this space in your head fill up with random things—some good, some bad, some helpful, and some not. (Nice plants in the garden, but also some weeds and deer ready to take over.) This is a tenuous situation at best.

3. You actively decide to fill this space in your head with positive inputs and refer to them often so they become ingrained. (You have very nice and well-tended plants in the garden, and you are out there EVERY SINGLE DAY making sure no weeds appear.) *This is what you want.*

For all you non-gardeners who still don't get it, the message is that you have to manage your thoughts (add good thoughts, remove or seek to minimize the bad ones, and maintain some focus on this process) every single day until you complete your treatment.

As for the metaphor, my garden was doing fantastic when we left for vacation, and it even received a lot of water while we were gone, but no one tended the garden, so things got a little bit out of control. Decent overall conditions but not a great result because it was not managed at a critical time.

WATCH WHAT GOES IN YOUR HEAD

If you till a garden and don't plant anything, weeds will show up almost immediately (at least in my garden). It's exactly the same with your cancer headspace. Let's say you aren't purposeful in what you allow to flow through your head and into your cancer headspace, especially right after diagnosis. You will likely end up with many worries and fears that aren't productive or helpful to you. Some examples might include the following:

- Concerns about survival rates for your type of cancer

- Fears about pain and discomfort during treatment
- Worries about how you can maintain your personal and professional commitments during treatment
- Fear that treatment won't be effective
- Doubts about the treatment itself
- Concern about losing your hair or overall appearance
- Recent negative experiences others have had with cancer or cancer treatment

I can tell you that these negative thoughts are all 100% useless and won't help you one bit, but you already know that. It's probably a natural inclination to think this way, however—at least at first. What's worse, many people who are trying to be helpful or even empathize with you will come up with questions or comments that trigger those thoughts. Some examples might be:

- "I would be worried sick about losing my hair."
- "I heard from person X that the radiation is very painful. I feel bad for you."
- "I hope you don't fall too far behind at work. I can help you where you need."

These people are trying to plant weeds in your garden, probably not on purpose, but that is exactly what is happening. I think people indirectly push their fears on you when they say these things and aren't really trying to express negative thoughts. Cancer scares the crap out of most people, and that fear can sometimes come out through those types of comments. Recognize them for what they are, let them pass, and move on.

You are in control of your thoughts and how you react to every single thing presented to you. MAKE 100% SURE you start to use that power to your absolute advantage. It's the most important thing we will talk about. Similar to a foundation for a house, it has to be strong.

Developing Positive Cancer Headspace Strategies

These strategies are listed from easiest to hardest (at least for me). No, they aren't natural at first. I will tell you how I internalized them first, and then we can go through an example of how those strategies can work in practice.

How I Internalized Positive Cancer Headspace Strategies

Honestly, I struggled with internalizing a positive cancer headspace when I first started trying to employ these strategies. They weren't really presented to me in or designed in any organized fashion, but they "felt right."

Step 1: Catch the Negative Thoughts

I knew it wasn't helpful to think negative thoughts about my cancer fight. I wasn't very good at managing my thoughts and feelings, at least not at first. The way I managed to start the process of catching negative thoughts, at least initially, was first to recognize a negative thought and then scold myself by saying (to myself), "That's crap ! I can't think that way." Next time you have a negative thought, catch yourself and tell yourself, in your words, to cut it out. An example: I (of course) read up on the survival rates for my type of cancer; it wasn't good news: five-year rate in the 20s. As I read the information, I said to myself, "Stop it! That's not helpful."

The first step is being aware of how you are thinking. Take it off autopilot.

This is pretty easy once you start to pay attention, and it continues to get easier over time. The one really important thing is that you don't beat yourself up for having the thoughts. Initially, recognize the thoughts and work to stop them but don't add unproductive emotion to the situation by punishing yourself for thinking some of those things in the first place. If you are sick, you really don't need to be beaten up any more than you already are.

We will deal with the negative thoughts in a minute. Right now, your first task is to learn to catch these thoughts and recognize them. I think, somewhere, your mind is exploring all possibilities, and the negative thoughts show up as part of the process. You may have to parse every thought for a while. It's exhausting, *but do it anyway.*

Step 2: Keep Positive Thoughts and Turn Around Negative Thoughts

This step was harder for me. Honestly, I got tired of scolding myself for negative thoughts, so I figured out a way to turn it around. I thought the same unhelpful thoughts over and over until I did something to stop it. When you are hopped up on steroids after three days in the hospital and on the stick (IV) the whole time, you either figure something out or go crazy.

I simply replaced the negative thought with something more positive or at least neutral. Going back to our first example, when I would think, *My cancer has a five-year survival rate in the 20s*, I would add, *So what? I am a sample size of one, and I will be part of the 20%.* It could have easily been something like, *I am at a great hospital with experts in my type of cancer*, or *I am pretty healthy, so I should have a positive outcome from treatment.* There are probably ten or twenty statements you can use to replace any unhelpful thought. Find one that makes sense to you. IMPORTANT: Go over the positive statements so many times that you can't think of the negative thought by itself without the positive response following.

Here are some ideas to spur add-on positive thoughts:

- Recalling others' successful treatments
- Realization of all of the people who are ready to support you during treatment
- Appreciation of all the doctors, nurses, and medical support staff who are doing their best to help get you well
- Previous success at overcoming obstacles
- Your own toughness, determination, prior good health, etc.
- Your faith

Actively working to spur positive thoughts is also an exercise in practicing gratitude in the face of a tough challenge. Be grateful for all the work and effort going into getting you healthy again by all the people in your treatment team and all of your supporters.

Step 3: Don't Let Negative Influences In

As you go through the cancer process, you have a lot of information thrown at you—some pointed right at you. Other information is widely available and finds its way to you, while some information is delivered to you as you "look around" either passively or on purpose.

For everything presented to you during your cancer process, ask the question whether it's helpful or not. Is the information one more something to worry about, or is it useful and will help you get well?

Sorting whether information was helpful or not was a bit of a challenge for me and was also tiring at first. Thankfully, it became second nature in pretty short order once I realized what was happening. As you think through old or new information related to your diagnosis and treatment, think to yourself, *Is this helpful or not?* Going back to our example, when I thought, *Wow, the survival rate for my cancer is pretty low*, I should have immediately thought, *Helpful or not?* That would've allowed the thought either to be discounted in my mind, passed by entirely, or be attached to something more positive.

I'm not suggesting you should live in a dream world and ignore everything negative. Process all the information you receive, but if it's merely a rehash of some bad news you have already heard, judge it, recognize it, and let it go.

Apply this thinking to people and other inputs like TV, social media, web pages, etc. By now, you likely know who and what aggravates you. Use that knowledge to purposely ignore those inputs. Read and watch other things. Excuse yourself from conversations and situations that irritate you. Avoid people who upset you. Everyone gets some type of "free pass" for being a cancer patient; use it purposefully and often to manage your mental inputs. It's important. This of it like turning the noise down so you can find a few moments of peace.

YOUR CANCER HEADSPACE—HERE'S WHAT WORKED FOR ME

1. <u>Figure out where you are</u>. Do you already have a bunch of negative thoughts rolling around in your head? Are you a blank slate? Do you already have a strategy to manage your thoughts?

2. <u>Start to identify negative thoughts as they occur</u>. Each day, recall your day and think about the subject of your thoughts. Sort through all of the negative thoughts each day. Don't give them energy; simply record them in your mind. Over time, transition this process to become something of an ongoing evaluation in your head. Remember, the easiest time to kill a negative thought is right after it occurs for the first time.

3. <u>Review the negative thoughts you recorded and IMMEDIATELY add a positive thought</u> (to replace it or append to the negative thought or worry). Work through all of the negative thoughts every day until you get the management of your cancer headspace under YOUR ACTIVE CONTROL. Again, it can feel exhausting, but do it anyhow.

4. <u>If you journal your negative thoughts, cross them out so you can still read them</u>. It's important to acknowledge the negative thoughts, but it's essential to journal your new, positive thoughts right behind them, preferably at the same time you are writing down the negative ones.

5. <u>Be aware of "Bad Weather."</u> Pay attention to how and what people are saying to you, and evaluate whether or not it is beneficial or supportive for you. Ban people who aren't helpful. (Yes, I am 100% serious.) Also, ban information that creates extra worry.

    a. Review conversations from each day that created stress. First, define some of the triggers (words, topics, etc.) that caused stress. Then, transition to catching these triggers within the conversations as they occur and discount or work to eliminate exposure to them accordingly.

    b. Don't stick your head in the sand if you get bad news. Don't go looking for or give energy to things that add stress or worry and aren't part of your path to recovery. If you get bad news, step up and deal with it.

6. <u>Build your fence</u>. Practice recognizing negative or unsupportive thoughts and inputs (or people), and don't let them in.

   a. Some examples might be reading things that focus on cancer hardship and worrying about whether treatment will work.

   b. This goes for people too. If specific people give you added stress in how they act (they create extra worry) or in how they relate to your treatment (constantly recall examples of people who had tough cancer journeys), then tell them to go away or tell your advocate to have them go away (nicely). Let them know that how they are communicating with you is adding unneeded stress.

7. <u>React slower</u>. If you are anything like me, your brain reacts as quickly as possible to pretty much anything or to at least form an opinion. To the extent you can, slow down your reaction, and become much more measured in your response to anything having to do with your cancer process. Being over-excited at bad or good news isn't always the best.

8. <u>Leverage mindfulness</u>. If you can, mindfulness and meditation are ways to slow things down, especially after you are first diagnosed. Taking these moments to "catch your breath" can be immensely valuable.

This chapter is foundational and will make all of the rest of the strategies much easier to implement as you move ahead. Take the time needed to get these concepts implemented for your situation. Grab a notebook and take notes, markup the margins in this book, and discuss with friends—whatever learning strategy will get you the best result in implementing the ideas discussed in this chapter.

Get yourself together—however you can do it.

4

TREATMENT—HOW TO ADVOCATE FOR YOURSELF

You are responsible to yourself, to love yourself,
to care for yourself, and to help yourself.

—Akiroq Brost

Newsflash: you are probably one of ten, twenty, or a hundred patients seen each day by the different members of your treatment team. You need to recognize the reality of the situation and act accordingly. That means you better learn to advocate for yourself. It's also 100% required for the next strategy for managing your treatment: Studied Indifference. Advocacy (and questioning) are the core tenets of the "studied" part of "Studied Indifference." That's a preview of the next chapter, but don't skip ahead now. ☺

If you aren't comfortable advocating for yourself, be honest and either

1. Push yourself to do it. (It may be uncomfortable but do it anyhow.)

2. Find someone you trust to advocate for you, and have them read Chapter 10.

Whatever you do, <u>DO NOT</u> leave THIS exact moment without figuring out how you will advoacte for yourself or have help in having it done for you. There are two rules for an advocate: it can't be anyone from your treatment team, and it has to be done in person.

You Were There When It Happened?

When I was a kid, I played outside a lot. I would get the usual bumps and bruises that come with playing outside with dogs, sticks, bikes, etc. Occasionally, my mom or dad would ask about a particularly ugly bruise or cut I had incurred during my outside explorations. Many times, I had no idea where I got the injury; it had simply happened when I was playing and wasn't particularly painful.

On the occasions I couldn't identify the injury's origin, my dad would invariably ask, "Were you there when it happened?" Yes, it was a witty comment meant to be funny, but it perfectly illustrates a VERY important point. You are likely the ONLY person present for every procedure, test, and scan during your cancer process.

So, pay attention to what is happening to you because it's very important that you use or relay this knowledge as you advocate for yourself or have someone advocate for you. Many people keep a journal to keep track of things. Your medical chart will get pretty fat if you have a long treatment process like mine. Make sure <u>you</u> take ownership of recalling everything that was done to you. The best way to do this is to write down everything.

An Extreme Lesson on Advocating for Yourself: My "Smartest Doctor" Story

I was "handed off" three times during my diagnosis and treatment. I started with a surgeon, then transitioned to a chemo doctor, and finally finished treatment with a radiation doctor. Honestly, I lucked out with my first two doctors, but even though I had great luck on the first two handoffs, I didn't leave anything to chance with the last. By then, I was a LOT more engaged in my treatment and unwilling to be on autopilot. My treatment was fabulous across the board, but I was always engaged when it was time.

I started with my general doctor. He referred me to The James Cancer Hospital at The Ohio State University. He wasn't sure it was cancer to start (allegedly), but he put me in the system there just in case, I guess. (Maybe he knew already.) I was referred to a great surgeon who ran the resident program at the time. He had a ton of pull and was a wizard with a scalpel. Plus, he was a great guy. Once the surgeon was done with me, I was referred to a very well-known T-cell cancer specialist (there aren't very many of them). I suppose there wasn't much choice because I had a rare type of cancer, and he was one of the top specialists in the US for my type of cancer—plus, he was already in the same hospital. Again, it was another good and lucky break for me.

So, it was time for another handoff when my surgeries and chemo were done. I met with my T-cell cancer doctor with my wife. He decided to pass me over to a radiation doctor. There were probably a lot of different radiation specialists who could do what I needed to have done—it wasn't super complicated. At least, it seemed that way as I understood it. As we discussed the referral, my T-cell cancer doctor told me there were a few different people who could do the radiation I needed. He named several, and, of course, I had never heard of any of them. I told him I wanted the "smartest one" of the bunch. Yes, I actually asked for the smartest doctor. My wife died (not literally) of embarrassment and looked at me very sternly after I made my request. My doctor laughed nervously. I simply stayed quiet. It was, at least for me, kind of a surreal moment.

The thing is, I was 100% serious. I wanted the smartest doctor. By this time, not much in my cancer fight was routine, so I wanted another really smart person on my side. Most importantly, I wasn't afraid to ask. In other words, I was advocating for myself.

Look, anyone who makes it through medical school and the additional training needed to become an oncologist has to be pretty smart. As with any profession, however, some doctors are simply smarter than others. Some are genius smart, and others were the last ones admitted to med school and maybe graduated at the bottom of their class. Some are simply better at their jobs or have had the capacity to understand more things or the same number of things better—that was the type of doctor I wanted.

I think it matters a lot because there can be a ton of gray areas in your diagnosis and treatment. Boy, did I find that out several times with "possibly" serious stuff. Intelligent doctors can look at the whole picture, take some strange lab results, and put them in a reasonable perspective. The longer your treatment continues, the more your body gets out of whack. Having someone who can calmly look at odd test results and give a confident assessment, good or bad, is key. It also reduces your stress, a lot. Good docs let you know, either directly or indirectly, when you should feel concerned too—no wishy-washy middle ground, but instead honest opinions based on experience that come pretty quickly. In my opinion, they are usually confident for a good reason; they are smart.

The Point of the Story: Advocate for Yourself

The point is to advocate for yourself and ask for the best doctors, along with the best of everything. It may not work out 100%, but at least ask. Don't treat it like the NFL draft, but do your homework. Ask for the smartest doctors, do some background checking by asking questions about the ones on your shortlist who are available, and decide on the best one for you. Also, ask the nurses—they *always* know. And, most importantly, don't be afraid to hurt someone's feelings by asking for what you feel you need. It doesn't mean you have to be demanding or behave rudely. It means being respectful and direct with your requests.

More Advocacy: Ask Questions; It Doesn't Matter That You Aren't a Doctor.

You are the expert of you. Don't forget that.

I will say it again—you are the expert of you. You are also the number one protector of yourself. Ask questions. I don't care if you struggled to pass the sixth grade; ask questions about whatever you don't understand. Keep asking questions until you understand whatever you are asking about—on your terms. It matters on two levels:

1. You need to make sure you understand exactly what is happening to you and what follow-on effects (good or bad) are possible.

2. You will feel much more confident in your ability to handle whatever treatment you will be put through if you fully understand the process—even if it will be very tough.

The broader point is that you are giving someone the go-ahead to poison or irradiate you (or worse), so you should probably ask a few questions—why questions (why am I getting this type of chemo), open-ended questions (what are possible complications), etc. *You will find that the MORE questions you ask, the more confident you will feel.*

You may not like the answers, but you will be less likely to feel surprised, worried, or upset later in the treatment cycle. As you go through this process, get all of your questions out, think of questions AHEAD OF TIME, and WRITE THEM DOWN. You will forget many of your questions when the doctor comes if you don't write them down right when you think about them. Remember the part about getting a journal? You should probably go do that now if you haven't already.

Be part of the treatment plan and understand it 100%. In this area, 95% is a failing grade. Sorry. Get additional medical opinions if you are not comfortable with your doctor. If you do this, gather all your medical records ahead of time to expedite the process.

Advocating for yourself doesn't only apply to doctors; do the work and research, and then at least ask for the best of everything: the best docs, the best medicines, and the best facilities. There are often choices of which you are not aware. Do some research, be engaged, have a view, listen to your doctors, and then ask for the best. Don't be a jerk about it, and be realistic about what may be possible, but at least ask.

Are There Really That Many Choices?

The short answer is yes. Some examples are

- Some rooms are on the same side as the hospital helicopter pad, and some aren't. It turns out Life Flights are an emergency and aren't always on a 9-5 schedule. See my blog at the back of the book for more on that. So you know, the rooms on the same side as the helicopter pad get to experience 100% of the noise of every helicopter landing, day or night.

- Some MRI machines are newer, bigger, and quieter than others. Maybe you can go to some other place in your health network to get to the bigger MRI machine for non-urgent scans, which is more comfortable and less stressful.

- Some medicines are optional, and some aren't. Ask if you have any optional medicines, then decide what you feel comfortable taking. Decide WITH your doctor. See my blog about my interaction with my nurse on my first day of chemo.

- Some inpatient nurse checks can be stretched. Being woken up every four hours at night is WAY better than every two hours, especially after three or four days of being an inpatient. This also applies to treatment schedules at times.

- Some treatments are even optional, so ask. I offer exactly zero advice on this. I only point out that you are probably NOT a doctor so discuss this in detail with your doctor. That said, I would suggest you do everything they suggest to get your cancer treatment done and cured on the first try.

- You can ask for specific doctors or specialists sometimes, so do it if you think it makes sense.

- You may be able to bring your own food into the hospital to eat. Ask.

You get the picture. Be an advocate for yourself. Don't be a pain in the butt (or bum if you're in England). Be nice. Be grateful. Be respectful, but at least ask for what you want; your care team will do their best to make it happen if you are nice about it. A great open ended question to ask: "Is there anything we can do to make (your issue) better?"

THE FINAL OUTCOME: WHY THE BEST DOCTORS?

It turns out it mattered for me, and, in my opinion, it probably always matters at least some.

My T-cell cancer doctor referred me to a great radiation doctor (after I asked for the smartest one). She was calm, very analytical, and really smart. I am pretty good at judging whether someone is smart, and she stood out as one of those people who was super bright but not arrogant while also being very helpful and patient. One thing you find out (at least I did) with all of the diagnoses and treatments is that there is a huge gray area in almost every part of treatment because each person is different.

Some of the gray area questions my doctors wrestled with were

- Should they surgically remove my tumor or treat it with chemo once they knew what it was?
- How many chemo treatments did I need to be fully cured of the lymphoma?
- Should I get a blood transfusion?
- What are the different ways the various scans can be interpreted?
- How should strange or inconsistent blood results be interpreted?

There are a ton of these gray areas that doctors, especially oncologists, sort out every single day. The smart(est) ones have enough functional understanding of the tests, scans, and their limitations. They have a good knowledge of all the interactions in your body to sort out the best approach for you and decide if something is really an issue.

Returning to my story, it was a bunch of back pain—really bad pain that was unusual for me. My radiation doctor sent me to get a scan of my back to see if there was "anything there"; that is, to check if the cancer had spread. The scan came back inconclusive from the radiologist. There MAY have been something there.

My radiation doctor looked at it for a few minutes and said, "I'm not impressed. We will watch it, but I don't think it's anything." There were four really important points here that did not go unnoticed by me:

1. She had an opinion and was willing to give it—no wishy-washy nonsense.

2. She could explain why she came up with her answer.

3. She wasn't stupid about the possibility that it COULD be something and made sure to monitor me for the weeks I was in her care to run the inconclusive MRI 100% to some conclusion, either way.

4. This lowered my stress level a few notches, not because of her diagnosis but mostly because she explained why she thought it was nothing.

For me, she was able to make a false alarm exactly that but smart enough to follow up on the possibility of trouble. That's why the smart doctor.

A Note on Sandbagging

What is sandbagging, you ask? Let me tell you. Here is a good definition that applies to our situation (bolding is mine): **hiding the** strength, skill, or **difficulty of something** or someone **early in an engagement**. Said another way, you may not be informed of the total course of your treatment or the difficulty of your treatment at the very beginning of the process. Your care team may still be sorting things out.

Now read only the bold parts.

Why am I telling you about this? It's easy. I suspect you might be sandbagged if you have a long journey ahead of you. Somehow, some way, you are probably not being told the whole story about your 100% complete course of treatment to protect you, to reduce your stress level, or because your doctor simply doesn't know yet. It's a hunch, but my cancer hunches are pretty good now.

Now, I am a reasonably bright person—good SAT scores, high scores on aptitude tests, the whole bit. In my first surgery, they opened me up, took a sample of the tumor, and sent it to pathology while I was still knocked out to see what it was so they could decide whether to cut out only the tumor or the tumor and some extra surrounding tissue if it was cancer. The pathology people were stumped while I was under, so they closed me back up, leaving the tumor right where it was.

So, I went back to my cancer surgeon after a few days so he could check on me. To my dismay, he told me that the pathology people weren't 100% done with the diagnosis. I asked him how long I'd need to heal before they could go back and cut out the tumor. He explained that he wasn't sure and they might let "the medicine" deal with the tumor.

During this, I thought that when the doctor said "medicine," that meant chemo, and I probably have cancer. They didn't have a definitive diagnosis at the time, and I expected they were still trying to sort out exactly if it was cancer, what cancer I had, and what they were going to do about it. I later found out this was 100% the case. They ended up sending my tissue to the National Institutes of Health (NIH) to confirm the diagnosis, and yes, they were right (smart docs on my side).

At the next visit, my surgeon and blood cancer doctor informed me that the tumor had to go. It turned out I got both another surgery AND chemo. Clearly, NOT a winning moment.

The point of the story is twofold:

1. Listen INTENTLY to what your doctors say. I could have easily not noticed the "medicine" comment. I knew then I was in trouble, but it was also clear that they weren't exactly sorted on an approach for me at my follow-up visit. Remember when I told you that I pretty much knew a cancer diagnosis was coming? This is how.

2. Keep asking about the WHOLE treatment plan. Your doctors may not have it yet, and that's OK. Some cases are more challenging

than others. If they don't have a whole plan together yet, mentally prepare yourself for a long journey. It isn't necessarily bad; it simply means that your doctors have more sorting to do to get your whole plan together or that some steps depend on the outcome of others (*i.e.*, how many total chemo treatments you will end up having).

How to Advocate for Yourself—Here's What Worked for Me

1. <u>Ask questions</u>. If you don't understand something, ask. If the person answering your question doesn't have the answer, ask someone else to explain it. **GET AN ANSWER!** It's 100% important and vital in reducing your stress. It may be a procedure, a wait time, or a drug you are taking. Ask about it until you understand it. See my blog highlighting my conversation with the hospital pharmacist on my first day of chemo.

2. <u>Understand your treatment plan, inside and out</u>. What is happening? When is it happening? Where is it happening? Who is doing the treatment? Why is it being done? What bad things could happen? What are the possible side effects? Ask EVERY question you can think of.

3. <u>Push—respectfully, but push</u>. Ask for the best of everything: The best room, the best MRI tube, the best and smartest doctors, the best of everything. Don't be a jerk, but at least ask.

4. <u>Make friends, especially with your nurses</u>. It will be a huge surprise when you learn how many different people you will come in contact with at a hospital or treatment center. I probably saw a few hundred people during my adventure. THEY ALL KNOW SOMETHING ABOUT WHO OR WHAT OPTIONS ARE "BETTER." Ask; some will tell you nothing, others will tell you everything they know. If you want to know who or what the best of something is—ask EVERY SINGLE PERSON you come in contact with. At a minimum, you will get some ideas on where to look.

5. <u>Keep notes</u>. Some days the doctors and the nurse practitioners looking after me blew through the room like the wind. I was a little interesting to them to start with (with my odd disease presentation), but after a while, not so much. You WILL forget a bunch of questions you had for the docs, so write them down so you can review them when they show up. Review your questions with a friend or advocate to make sure you didn't leave anything out.

6. <u>Understand your schedule</u>. Daily, weekly, monthly if needed. I was "point to pointed" or "sandbagged," as I suspect that most people with long treatments are. That means you are told the next step or two only for your whole treatment. This may be for your whole treatment plan or can also be done for a long day filled with a lot of procedures (think back to my first day in).

THIS PART IS IN ALL CAPS FOR A REASON: IT'S IMPORTANT.

IF YOU FEEL LIKE YOU ARE 100% OVERWHELMED, FEEL DEPRESSED, OR THINK YOU COULD HURT YOURSELF, ASK FOR PROFESSIONAL HELP. TELL THE FIRST PERSON YOU CAN ON YOUR CARE TEAM, YOUR FAMILY, OR YOUR FRIENDS, AND TELL THEM YOU NEED HELP RIGHT NOW.

EVEN IF YOU TALK TO A PROFESSIONAL ONLY ONCE TO GET YOUR HEAD RESET, DO IT.

5

TREATMENT—STUDIED INDIFFERENCE

All things are ready if our mind be so.

—William Shakespeare, *85/-7*

I struggled with coming up with a good name for this concept. As mentioned previously, it does not mean you are indifferent to your diagnosis, treatment, or anything else during the process. What it does mean is that once you have done the work to understand your treatment, exactly what is happening, and what can possibly go wrong (the "studied" part), you *decide* to become indifferent to the process as it occurs. Sit back, let it happen, and focus on what <u>you</u> can do to get better.

There's a vital distinction between simply being indifferent about treatment and actively studying everything about your treatment with the INTENT of developing enough confidence to release stress to the point of indifference when the treatment is underway. This is your goal.

It means you are doing your homework, letting go of the stress, and letting the professionals do what they need to do. It means if you get a bad side effect that was already explained to you, plan for the possibility, accept it and manage through it. If something goes sideways, outside the things you already considered, you reengage fully, understand what is happening, understand the revised plan, and then let *it* happen.

Trying to manage your response as things happen (or go sideways) in your treatment can be very difficult. I found it's best to apply the principle of planning reactions to possible negative side effects ahead of time and being fully informed about your treatment and possible issues.

This approach is basically an adaptation of the E+R=O (Event plus Response equals Outcome) concept attributed to Jack Canfield. E+R=O means that while you don't always control the "E," you DO control the "R" and, as such, have a great influence on the "O". The Studied Indifference concept is easier if you use the E+R=O process <u>as your treatment is decided or planned, NOT as it happens</u>. We work ahead to determine as many possible events as possible and preplan our responses to those events for the best possible outcomes for our treatment.

Your treatment may contain some roadblocks and surprises. Even everyday items can become a challenge. The time to decide how to react to these obstacles is before they even happen. How is this possible? It is possible because before you agree to any treatment, you need to ask questions and a lot of "what ifs" to understand all possible bad things that can happen during treatment. This allows you to mentally prepare and, more importantly, decide how to respond in the most positive way possible to any treatment complications or roadblocks *before* they occur.

STARTING TO FIGURE IT OUT: THE BEGINNINGS OF STUDIED INDIFFERENCE

I stumbled into this approach during my treatment. In all honesty, I was kind of forced into it. I first considered the Studied Indifference approach during the first part of my journey. It all started, though, with the fine needle aspiration.

I was referred to the James Cancer Center at The Ohio State University by my general doctor because I had a tumor about the size of half an egg (cut longwise) on the back of one of my legs—near my hamstring. I saw the cancer surgeon for the first time, and he was a bit perplexed by the tumor. Honestly, he wasn't really sure what to make of it. It was in a really weird spot and didn't fit any predetermined cancer presentation. He was happy to cut it out (recommended because it was growing) but wanted to know exactly what it was before doing anything. If it was cancer, they would cut the tumor out with a bunch of nearby tissue to get all of it; if it wasn't, they would chop the tumor out and not take the extra tissue.

During that first visit, my surgeon couldn't quite determine what it was and wanted pathology to help sort it out. At this point, I was starting to get a little nervous. He called the medical school and asked one of the pathology doctors who also taught there to come right over. (My surgeon was great and had the good pull to make things happen quickly.)

About twenty minutes after the call from my surgeon, the pathology doctor arrived with a small "house call" bag—he was an earnest guy, older, maybe in his early 60s, no-nonsense, and upright with a deep voice. Two budding and very serious interns filed in after him—I was a pretty interesting case, after all. He said they intended to get a few samples of the tumor but then dropped the bad news; no numbing for the procedure (it's bad for the sample). So they prepped to stick my tumor (me) with a pretty long needle, which they would have to do several times to get three samples for analysis—one for the doctor and each intern.

The doctor first poked the needle into my leg and tumor, and it hurt, a lot. Then he started "scraping," which really hurt—it brought tears to my eyes. While this was happening, my wife was watching the drama from the corner—not really watching what was happening but watching my reaction to it—and told me to look at her to get through it. The first intern was next to take a stab at me. He poked near the edge of the tumor this time, and the poke felt about the same, but his cell scraping method, frankly, sucked. He had to scrape for 20–30 seconds to get his cells. After noticing how flushed and sweaty I was at this point, my wife finally looked at the procedure in progress for the first time. Bad idea.

The next thing I heard was the pathology doctor asking, "Ma'am, are you OK?" She wasn't; she doesn't do blood or needles, so the scene wasn't a great combo. Her face was ghostly white. Needless to say, she ended up looking at the wall for the remainder of the procedure.

Despite the drama and not wanting to waste a good training case, intern number two stepped up. She poked, scraped to get her harvest, and wrapped up in about half the time of the first intern. My wife remained staring at the wall and, thankfully, didn't pass out. My leg really, really hurt, however. Looking back, it was a quick procedure, but it felt like it took forever—for both my wife and me.

When I thought about it later, it was an excellent teachable moment for me. This procedure had to happen as a step in the process. I could fight it, yell, scream, whine, complain, or ask for another approach— or I could let it happen. I had not yet learned the indifference part of Studied Indifference as this all happened pretty fast—that realization would come later.

It was, however, my first lesson in Studied Indifference. The procedure was something that had to happen. It was well explained (easy to understand, so I didn't have to advocate or study too much), short in duration (limited developed patience or toughness required), and a procedure where, if I tensed or moved or fought it physically (*i.e.*, wasn't indifferent), it either would have caused more damage or would not have resulted in a viable sample. I never realized it at the time, but it was a great lesson to set a base for the future of developing a mental model to deal with every treatment.

The Final Straw: Being Forced into Studied Indifference for Good

(Mostly paraphrased from my blog post)

I got to the hospital at 6 AM to start my first chemo round (four scheduled days inpatient that ended up being five days), and they told me they didn't have a bed for me on the hematology floor. I got as upset as someone could be at 6 AM, tried to help the hospital solve the problem, and finally decided there was NOTHING I could do. NOTHING. It was quite a revelation for someone who tries almost every day to make things happen. I tried to find patience at that point but was mad, scared, and impatient all at once. So I went for some coffee. I returned a while later, and they found me a room.

I got settled in my room around 8:30 AM. Soon afterward, a nurse arrived to check my vitals; I was ready to go. Ready like right now. When the IV was put in, she told me that she was waiting for the doctor to issue the orders to the pharmacy. Being mindful of wanting total knowledge of what was happening to me, I asked the nurse what was in my chemo cocktail. She listed the ingredients and what she thought each ingredient did. It wasn't a great explanation. So, I asked to discuss it with my doctor or a pharmacist to get a solid description of the drugs in my chemo cocktail (some advocacy and some curiosity on my part). Having now gained a reputation for demanding knowledge, the pharmacist showed up with a HUGE pile of paper and patiently explained each drug. That gave me a good understanding of the chemo drugs and all the other drugs given during chemo. They passed that test, so I decided to let them "poison" me. (I know, a harsh description for a life-saving compound.) These few instances, from my first day as an inpatient, represent my first real bout of advocacy.

(Remember the lesson about sandbagging? Here we go. ☺)

Soon thereafter, I was told I needed a heart ultrasound to ensure I had a healthy heart as some of the chemo drugs can cause heart conditions. It took two hours to schedule these tests I knew nothing about. I suspect the nurses knew but were waiting on those orders as well.

My heart was deemed OK, so it began a waiting game for the chemo bags to arrive. During the wait, my nurse told me I needed a PICC line—they can't (or don't) use a regular IV for chemo. I didn't even know what a PICC line was at this point. It turns out a PICC line is a line with a long tube inserted about halfway up the inside of your bicep and fed to a major artery somewhere in your chest.

First, nobody told me about this ahead of time, and those nurses (very specialized) would be in "later." Around 3 PM, two nurses rolled in, both a barrel of monkeys—hilarious to each other (and to me at this point). My questions started before they did. It was about a fifteen-minute interrogation on my part, after which I allowed them to insert the PICC line. They were great at their job, and it went without incident.

With the PICC line in, I was ready to start my first round of chemo—or so I thought. The nurse casually mentioned they usually start chemo in the morning, so you don't get discharged at night. But I was OK getting discharged at night and urged them to get started. About the same time, the nurse practitioner (NP) sauntered in (about 5:00 PM) and asked if I had had the bone marrow draw yet. Nope. I was pissed—super pissed and entering a FULL meltdown. I hadn't expected this—the PICC line, the ultrasound, or the long delay in getting a room. It had been a ridiculous day that started at 6 AM.

Technically, the bone marrow draw isn't required, but with my type of cancer, they like to check it to make sure it's clear before treatment begins. If it's not clear, it could be a much bigger adventure ahead. I figured it was a smart idea to allow it, but it would be TOMORROW. After asking questions for about fifteen minutes, the NP said she'd do it first thing in the morning.

At about 9 AM the next day, the NP, a cart full of supplies and an assistant showed up. She injected me with something to "take the edge off" before drilling into my back to get her sample. (The procedure feels like someone rattling your bones FROM THE INSIDE. Unsettling, at best.)

Chemo was finally ready to start at 11:00 or so on day 2. But first, I had to swallow a whole pile of pills—10–12 pills, I think (at least the first day). With EACH ONE, I asked, *What is it? What does it do? Do I have to take it? What are the side effects?* The nurse kept rolling her eyes, but near the end of the interrogation, we were joking about it. I opted against about four of the optional pills and agreed to take them only if needed.

I wish I had known then what I know now about Studied Indifference. My first few hours in the tank (hospital) were a mental disaster of my own making. I was all over the place mentally. I wasn't a good advocate at the time (I didn't understand the whole process and didn't study) and couldn't let go (I kept getting frustrated, and couldn't get to indifference). My guess is some of it was stress, but some were because I hadn't developed the mental skill to sort through an incredibly busy thirty-six hours.

It's a long story, I know, but it forced me to learn the concept of Studied Indifference—pound away at the questions, know the plan, and then sit back and let the professionals do their job.

BE A PATIENT PATIENT

At some point after that first day, I purposefully decided to be patient with the process. I wanted to do what I could to keep things on schedule, but also be patient. Being patient gets easier for three reasons:

1. You know how things work and how slow things can be. With perspective, I thought about the fact that they were poisoning me on purpose and wanted to be careful.

2. You get better at being patient; keep practicing. (Insert joke about being an actual patient here.)

3. You feel so crappy that nothing is a rush. Here's to hoping you don't land here as I did. (Thankfully, I found a positive way to think about anything.)

I wasn't nervous about anything they gave me via IV or pill or about any procedure they had to do on me because I asked enough questions to get settled with the medicine or procedure before they did it. It's tough to relax when you have these treatments and are receiving some serious drugs. By eliminating all of your uncertainty (or as much as possible) about what is being done, however, you have the best chance possible to be relaxed (and indifferent) as treatments progress.

VERY IMPORTANT: *Be very respectful and polite when you ask these questions. Your treatment team will be your best advocate and supporter, and in the end, they are there to help you.*

Treat them with the respect they deserve.

To be 100% honest, I wasn't perfect on this score. I got into it pretty good with an NP who wanted to force me into having an optional but "highly recommended" blood thinner. She couldn't convince me I needed it. I was reasonably fit and young with no history to indicate the need for the medicine, so I said no thanks—my body, my rules. She left unimpressed, and I never saw her again during my treatment. In general, hold your fire with your care team; it's really the best approach. It wasn't my finest hour, I suspect.

STUDIED INDIFFERENCE—HERE'S WHAT WORKED FOR ME

1. <u>Wear your treatment team out with questions, then let go</u>. Make sure you ask every question you can think of regarding your treatment for the (day/week/month) and what COULD happen, both good and bad. Don't let anyone poke you, hook you up to an IV, take a scan, or give you medicine unless you know why you are getting it, you understand, and you agree. Wear the doctors and nurses out with questions. Without this, you won't be able to let go of the stress and become indifferent. Once you are out of questions and understand your treatment, let go and let it happen.

2. <u>If something unexpected happens, re-engage, ask all the questions you need to understand the situation and medical response, and then let the professionals do their work</u>. Treatment is rarely a straight line—know that complications may be coming and be ready to re-engage, with a level head, to sort out the situation and seek to get back to a full understanding of the, now revised, path forward.

3. <u>When things get bogged down, delayed, extended, canceled, rescheduled, or changed, decide—AHEAD OF TIME—to learn</u>

to say "whatever." It will happen. It's not productive to complain or get angry. It won't help your treatment. Step in to advocate for yourself with your care team where needed, and make sure it's productive and respectful. Have an alternative time killer ready: a book, video, person to call, or whatever you can pick up to pass the time.

4. <u>The real world and its challenges will continue to roll on while you are in treatment.</u> Again, think through things AHEAD of time where you can. ASK for help, and then let go. If you miss a hair appointment or the dog doesn't get dinner one night, it's OK. Acknowledge things will happen, and you will be able to manage through them. *IMPORTANT: If you are feeling overwhelmed, ask for help RIGHT AWAY.*

5. <u>Be respectful of your treatment team at all times.</u> –THIS IS IMPORTANT—they are YOUR team (and your only team). Be good to them, and as Jerry McGuire says, "Help them help you."

6. <u>Be patient. Figure out the best way to do this for you.</u> All of my suggestions center around positive distractions or time killers that I used. Not that anyone needs any more advice on how to kill time but here goes:

    a. Watch funny movies, shows, or YouTube clips.

    b. Read something faith-based: the Bible, a book, a blog, etc.

    c. Meditate if you know how.

    d. Read something with a positive outcome: the girl gets the guy, the team wins the game, etc. NO EXCEPTIONS on the positive part.

    e. Watch documentaries on positive or neutral things—nothing about murders, drug dealers, etc.

    f. Watch comedies. Norman Cousins, an American political journalist, author, professor, and world peace advocate, laughed his way to health in the 1960s.

    g. Sleep.

    h. Call friends.

i.   Blog. (See mine at the end of this book. It's at least a *little* funny.)

j.   Email friends.

k.   Delete old computer or email files.

l.   Read self-improvement books.

m. Listen to happy music.

n. Pet your dog or cat.

6

TREATMENT—TOUGHNESS RESPONSE

If you are going through hell, keep going.
—Winston Churchill

When you have cancer, you had better either be tough or be able to call on your personal strength to become tough—like right now. You will be challenged through your physical and mental journey, and you had better be ready. By reading this book and getting yourself "ready"—or thinking about it—you are already on your way to being able to respond to physical and mental challenges in a positive and productive way and with a Toughness Response.

The number of ridiculous things a doctor can order to be done to your body is astounding. Some of them hurt—a lot. Some are disconcerting, like the required lead tubes surrounding the radioactive stuff they inject you with for some scans. More importantly, as you progress through treatment, you might get to the point where your mental capacity to manage yourself and control your reactions to stress, pain, or discomfort is severely limited. You also still probably have things to do in your everyday life that have to get done. It's at that exact time that you will need to connect to your physical or mental toughness either to push through certain portions of your treatment or to be able to work on the things you need to have done.

In both cases, the challenges, either mental or physical, may not have been fully anticipated. These unexpected challenges will happen; the important thing is how you respond to them. That's why we are focused on a toughness response. You will seek not to react with fear or weakness; you will choose, on purpose, to respond with strength and toughness. Yes, it's a choice—100%. Make the decision and commit to that approach. Decide to be tough first: both mentally and physically.

In this book, I talk about having a structured approach to managing these challenges through your treatment process. This strategy is mostly process driven. You work ahead of your treatment, stay ahead of the mental challenges, know what physical challenges could come up, and work to manage them as much as possible ahead of time.

Mental challenges show up mostly as fatigue on three levels:

1. You are sick of being sick, mentally worn out by the daily challenge of being sick.

2. You are tired of managing all of the details required to manage your part of the treatment process, *i.e.*, process fatigue.

3. You encounter some unexpected change in your condition or treatment that tries to push you off of your process, *i.e.*, bad news.

4. We will address each of these challenges independently.

Mental Challenges

It's crucial to think proactively to stay ahead of most of the known or likely mental challenges in your treatment. You can do this by proactively following some of the strategies in this book. Each of the different mental challenges will require you to plan ahead or react in a different way.

Mental Challenge 1: Sick of Being Sick

I certainly got to a point where I was "sick of being sick." I was worn down, tired, and stressed. You get the picture. Not every cancer patient may get to this point, especially if they have a relatively short treatment process. You may be there perpetually if your cancer is very advanced. It's a different experience for everyone.

There are a bunch of different reasons you arrive at this place in your thinking. Maybe you missed a big event, or you tried to do something you really wanted or needed to do but couldn't. Or perhaps you looked in the mirror and didn't recognize the person staring back. Whatever the trigger, something pushed you to the point where you realized or decided that you were sick of being sick.

When this point comes, let it happen. Give yourself a mental break because you will feel more mentally fatigued if you fight it. Stand back, recognize where you are mentally, and do one of two things:

Ask for help or talk to someone.

Give yourself a break. Be OK with the frustration temporarily, but set a time you plan to reengage and process it. It's like taking a vacation from your stress. You can get wound up sometimes. So every once in a while, you simply have to let go. This is a few hours type of thing. You need to reengage purposefully after you have given yourself a mental break.

I never had the opportunity to plan for this type of fatigue, but you may be able to. Tell your advocates that if the time comes when you need to "check out" mentally for a few hours, you will need them with you to help you stay distracted, calm, or whatever. They should also be the ones to help you "check back in" to your process. If you feel like you can't reengage, ask for help right away.

Mental Challenge 2: Treatment Detail Mental Fatigue

It sounds complicated, but this means that you get to a point where you get mentally exhausted at keeping up with all that is going on each day with your treatment. I had so many things going on at one point, right after exiting surgery and when I started chemo, that I could hardly keep up: wound care, chemo plans, blood draws, bone marrow draws, PICC lines, scans, biopsy reports, etc. It was crazy, and it wore me out mentally.

With this type of fatigue and in cases where your understanding of your treatment plan is barely out ahead of your actual treatment, *you have to push through*, either by yourself or with help. I don't have a better answer. You really don't want to get to the position where your understanding of what is next is chasing what is actually happening.

I can tell you from experience that it will all slow down in your head at some point. It can be a huge volume of information to process initially. As we mentioned before, processing your treatment plan is the key to reducing the stress you are experiencing during each treatment. I can also tell you that the hospital won't likely slow treatment down because you haven't mentally processed all of it yet.

Later in your treatment, it may be possible to build a longer-term understanding of your treatment plan. If you get to that point and need to disengage for a few days, you are still ahead of what is happening. When you feel stronger, push your treatment team to understand your treatment plan details further out into the future. After several weeks, I did manage to get to this point.

Mental Challenge 3: Unexpected Complications

There may be some other unforeseen mental hurdles or quickly developing mental challenges you have to deal with. Some examples might be unexpected treatment complications, pain worse than was expected or a change in routine or treatment plan, or some unexpected outside "regular life" issue like a sick child or pet. In short, this is something that creates stress you did not anticipate.

These circumstances simply turn into another "get yourself together" moment where you have to choose—*on purpose*—to address the new information, reengage mentally, and figure out what to do next. The best advice I can give here is to do this on YOUR timeline.

This isn't a case where you can simply disengage. If it's new information and you need to form a response, do it on your schedule, where possible. Obviously, if you are being rushed into emergency surgery, that's one thing, but, in my experience, there is almost always time to process things before deciding on a response.

Here is a real-life example:

A Short Complications Story

The day after Christmas, I got a fever during one of my chemo cycles. For people not in chemo treatment, a fever is generally an uninteresting situation. For a chemo patient, it is a red alert to the medical staff. When your immune system is severely depressed, it turns out that the last thing you need is an infection. It can be very serious.

I was over the fever "red line" (the temperature where you had to IMMEDIATELY go to the hospital to get intervention). My wife took my temperature a few times over the course of ninety minutes or so, and there was no doubt I was over the line.

The problem was that I didn't want to go to the hospital. I wasn't mentally ready to deal with it.

I KNEW I had to go; I simply wasn't ready. So, I waited a bit. It wasn't like me sitting on my couch an extra thirty minutes was going to make a huge difference in my treatment when I got back to the hospital, so I took the time. I needed a few minutes to sort things in my head because I knew it was going to be pretty crappy to be back in the tank, and it was. When I got there, they cleaned out the antibiotic cabinet, gave me some narcotics, and held me for a few days—in time to start my next chemo round. It was awful.

The moral of the story that is when these things come up, you decide to do the right thing (in my case, go to the hospital), but take a moment or two to process what is going on and get mentally reset so you are ready for what's coming at you.

One final note on the mental challenges you face. As you get further into your treatment—and it certainly was my experience—you might not be all there mentally. Sometimes you know or sense your loss of mental faculty (for me, I felt "slow"). At other times, you have no clue. In my situation, this indicated an approach that started with a purely physical and defiant mental state that could become more rational based on how well my brain was functioning at the time. Said another way, you decide to tough out the challenge in front of you FIRST, then start to deconstruct the issue and develop a better mental approach if and when you are mentally able.

Physical Challenges

As for the physical challenges, they can often be surprising and worse or different than you expected. Even though the mental side of managing yourself is, in my opinion, the most important, it is critical to face physical challenges as well. Physical challenges primarily come in two forms:

1. Chronic conditions: Daily nausea, headaches, pains, and the like, usually in the form of some type of pain or discomfort that is mostly present but not acute.

2. Acute but mostly temporary pain: Things like pain from surgical sites, radiation burns, extreme constipation, or other short-term but very painful or uncomfortable conditions.

Again, we will address each of these conditions independently.

Depending on your treatment and type of cancer, you will likely experience discomfort or pain during the treatment regime. Some of the pain and discomfort will be unexpected or worse than you thought it might be when the treatment plan was explained to you. As we discussed, some physical pain will be chronic, and some pain will be acute. You have to deal with each of these types of physical pain separately.

Treatment-Induced Chronic Pain

Your treatment may cause you chronic pain in the form of nausea, constipation, headaches, burns, or other things. It's not surprising; if you did your homework, you knew these types of discomfort were possible.

The first time it comes up, every kind of discomfort is a reportable condition to your treatment team. For example, if you get nauseated, like was mentioned as a possible side effect of chemo, tell your treatment team when it first happens. They will gather more information about it to make sure it is something expected of your treatment. If you have the same condition, but it later gets worse, again, tell your treatment team so they can investigate more where needed. Help your team help you.

Once you have told your treatment team about these types of chronic discomforts and they have determined they aren't unusual and that they have given you whatever medicine they can give you to offset the discomfort, you need to make a decision. Are you going to whine or worry continually or give energy to the discomfort or are you going to decide, on purpose, to respond with toughness?

In these cases, it's really that simple. Just go.

Believe me, I parsed this ten ways to Sunday in my head as I was sick. I had nausea, crazy headaches, radiation burns, surgery pain—the whole package. I used different medicines to partially treat each of these conditions but rarely did they disappear fully. So, you get to the point where you can decide to let it take over your thinking, or you choose, on purpose, to recognize the discomfort and ride it out.

I became defiant. I wasn't going to let these types of things win. I wasn't going to allow these types of chronic conditions to stop me from doing what I could otherwise physically do. I intentionally decided to be mentally tough in response to this type of pain. If it wasn't a new medical issue (as determined by my doctors) and it wasn't life-threatening, I knew my only choice was to push through it.

This might not be a significant insight, but it's real life.

Acute Physical Pain Response

Not everybody will experience acute pain during their treatment, but I 100% believe that you have to be prepared and plan how to deal with it. Not every treatment plan includes this possibility, but, as with any medical process, things can change and cause unexpected issues. Sometimes, you know it's coming; sometimes, you don't.

I knew I would have some pain after my two leg surgeries. The incision was in a weird place (the back of my leg, over my hamstring), leaving me in a straight-leg brace for a while after each surgery. It wasn't great, but, honestly, it wasn't the most acutely painful thing I experienced—that would come later.

About a week after each inpatient chemo stay, my body would be at its lowest point physically. During that time, I had unbelievable constipation. Really, really, unbelievable constipation. There aren't enough superlatives to describe it accurately. On Wednesday or Thursday of those "low weeks," I would get bouts of stomach pain that were so bad that I would lay on my couch, curled up and sweating. They lasted about an hour each time it happened, sometimes a few times a day. It was awful. Worse yet, it wasn't something that I was specifically warned about, at least the possible severity of the issue.

The first time it happened, I dutifully called the nurse and asked for help. She gave the usual suggestions, all over-the-counter laxatives. None worked for me, not even close. So, I suffered and sweated through the pain through concentration, distraction, prayer, movement, and taking action. Maybe not literal action but by doing something that had a chance of relieving the pain.

Here are some of the strategies I used for these short-duration (one hour or less) very high-pain periods:

- Defiance—Mental state that I was not going to let this get to me.
- Concentration—I tried to read (pretty hard) or play solitaire (easier).
- Distraction—Watching something funny (this seemed to work the best).
- Prayer—Pray for some relief. I don't think I was doing it exactly right because I still was usually still in pain at the end of my praying. ☺ Asking for help seemed to provide some hope that things would get better sooner than if I hadn't asked for help.
- Taking Action—Calling my care team or having my wife look on the internet for possible solutions seemed to provide hope and a good distraction. It ultimately solved my problem.

Don't think it will be the case every time, but being determined to at least look for a resolution sometimes turns up an answer to relieve your pain. Make sure that whatever you do is under your care team's medical supervision.

Keep Working on the Problem

My wife can't stand to see anyone she loves feel pain. At times, she literally comes close to fainting (like she did with my first biopsy). When I was curled up on the couch, sweating, it drove her crazy not to be able to help me. She looked for ideas on the internet about how to fix my crazy constipation and called the nurses a few times a day but to no avail until she called a friend of ours who was an oncology nurse.

Now, don't get the wrong idea here. I don't advocate doctor or nurse shopping, but we were friends with this family for years, and the oncology nurse was already at my hospital and was super smart (studying for a Ph.D. at the time), so she wasn't going to recommend anything outside of good treatment standards. My wife explained my predicament, and the nurse friend gave my wife the name of an over-the-counter laxative that they have cancer patients use in extreme cases. She advised me to start with half of the bottle and go from there.

My wife rushed to the store to get the new laxative (it's over the counter, and no, I'm not naming it), came home, and I drank it down. I waited, and nothing happened for about thirty minutes. Then, all of a sudden, we had a "breakthrough." I was back to normal about an hour later. Good as new. I felt a million times better.

I later asked my regular nurses about taking this laxative. Some laughed, and some gave some pretty hilarious warnings about using it, but they universally said it was safe, but they didn't always prescribe it because the results can be a bit "aggressive."

It won't often work out this way with bouts of acute pain, but I think it perfectly illustrates the point that you have to *keep working on the problem* until you are through the pain or find a different, medically approved approach that works.

In both of the stories in this chapter, the mental or physical challenges were not always expected. This will happen. The important thing is how you respond to it. That's why we are focused on a toughness response. <u>You will seek not to respond with fear or weakness</u>; you will choose to respond with strength and toughness, and with a plan, <u>on purpose</u>.

Yes, it's a choice, 100%.

Make the decision and commit to that approach. Decide to be tough first—both mentally and physically. As you sort this out for your situation, if you need help, ask for it.

Mental Toughness Response—Here's What Worked for Me

<u>Confirm Your Foundation</u>—As we have mentioned, the most important foundational action you can take is to advocate for yourself. I know I'm repeating material from another chapter, but it is really the base you need to develop, to the best of your ability, your plan to deal with the mental challenges ahead.

- Know the path of your treatment plan and the associated timing.
- Know what parts of your treatment plan typically induce difficulties.
- Know what could go wrong. What are some possible complications?
- Ask, specifically, when you will be most tired or fatigued during your planned treatments.

<u>Build A Good List of Possible Diversions</u>—Build your list of "go to" diversions for when you become fatigued or stressed. Some examples are

- Prayer
- Reading
- Playing games on a tablet or phone

- Listening to music
- Watching videos (especially funny videos)
- Knitting
- Coloring Books
- Reiki or Chair Yoga

Defiance—Determine what your strategy is going to be when you experience times you simply have to push through. What is effective "self-talk" to get you to push through difficult mental periods? Some ideas on where to start are

- Recalling success in other mentally challenging situations
- Vivid movie scenes that demonstrate persistence, defiance, and determination of some other means of facing a challenge.

Reframe Your Focus—What can you do to simply focus on something else?

- Watch something inspiring
- Read
- Move
- Cook
- Nap
- Meditate
- Eat (healthy!)

Input Control—Decide, ahead of time, what you will allow yourself to consume on social media, TV, the internet, etc. As we would tell our kids, "make good choices."

- Say yes to funny or inspirational material
- Say no to depressing or other depressing material

Build your mental support team and have an accountability partner—If, at some point, you need to check out mentally for a few hours, you will need to have someone at the ready to bring you back "online." Know who that person is right now and ask them to be on standby and tell them what to tell you, if necessary.

Know where to turn. Know where—exactly—you will get professional help if needed. If you don't have a VERY clear answer to that question, work to get it sorted right away.

For an extra credit mental challenge—Go out when you look and feel your worst. I know, we spoke about how to deal with mental challenges and, at first, this simply seems like you are adding additional stress to your life but hear me out.

When you go out when you are looking and feeling bad, it turns out to be the ultimate form of acceptance. It doesn't mean that you like how you look or feel. It means that you truly accept it, and you can let go of the stress that comes with the worry of looking or feeling a certain way. It can be a very powerful means of developing mental toughness.

For me, this meant going out to the gym. Soon after I started my chemo treatment, I had no hair and skin that looked dry, scaly, and pasty. Overall, I looked like a ghost or someone ready to keel over and die. You get the picture. When I look back on it, the minute I decided to go out in public looking sickly was the moment I accepted where I was. I became willing to "simply go" to do whatever was needed to get better or live my day-to-day life.

Overall, know some mental challenges are coming and decide how you will respond positively to these and other unforeseen challenges. Win the battle between your ears before it starts. Get ready for challenges, right now.

PHYSICAL TOUGHNESS RESPONSE—HERE'S WHAT WORKED FOR ME

Confirm Your Foundation—As we have mentioned, the most important foundational action you can take is to advocate for yourself. As it relates to physical pain, you need to be able to answer the following questions:

- What physically happens during each procedure or step of my treatment?
- What physical challenges can those procedures generate for you?
- What are the common side effects of procedures or drugs being prescribed for treatment?

In short, the advocacy here is much more about the "hands-on" portion of your treatment and what possible pain the associated procedures can generate.

Have a Plan—Throughout your advocacy, you will have developed a good-sized list of possible physical side effects from your treatment. For each possible side effect, have a plan on how you will address it. Some examples:

- *Headaches*—Sometimes, during chemo, you can't take regular pain relievers and have to take narcotics instead. Know how you plan to handle this and whether you will simply have to develop a plan to work through headaches or deal with the side effects of another medicine.
- *Soreness*—Some examples might be radiation soreness, surgical soreness, or muscle soreness. Some sample responses:
  - Radiation soreness—use of creams or ointments as prescribed, certain types of clothes that feel cool to the touch, showers, or baths when allowed. For me, cool showers were very helpful.
  - Surgical soreness (positioning)—ask specifically about what positions or postures may be most beneficial in relieving or muting soreness. Find out what postures are not allowed and explore, purposefully, on your own. For me, it was simple: don't stretch the surgical area.

- o Muscle soreness—find out what you can and can't do concerning physical activity, then work on finding a massage or stretching regimen that helps. Since I had surgery on my leg and was in a straight leg brace for several weeks, I found that simply lying down without the brace actually allowed some of the muscles in my leg to relax.

- *Nausea*—Know what types of interventions your doctor recommends and where you can obtain these items if needed.

- *Other side effects mentioned by your care team*—Know how you can respond to other physical discomfort that may be a side effect of your treatment.

Distractions—What is your go-to list of distractions to reduce focus on physical pain? (See the list of distractions and focus-reframe ideas presented above.)

You have all the toughness strategies you need at this point, so get ready. Be on the lookout for the type of situations that may cause mental or physical distress, and sort your first line of response for both mental and physical pain. Actively look for trouble ahead so you can sort out how you can respond, now and with a clear head, if a challenging situation arises.

7

TREATMENT—APPLIED DETERMINATION

Determination is the wake-up call to the human will.

—Tony Robbins

T his concept is one of the most important we will introduce. It's the bridge between the chaotic, crazy life of treatment and an attempt to return to normalcy. It means you make your mind up to do something (determination) and then do it (applied). Applied determination isn't something that is necessarily done in real-time. (Decide now and do it now.) Why? Because you may not be in a position, either physically or mentally, at any given moment to do what it is you set out to do.

If you decide to do something far ahead of time, however, and you prepare yourself accordingly, AND you apply your determination to do it, three really good things happen:

1. *You get whatever it is done and complete.* It may be a small thing, like making lunch for your kids, going out to the grocery store, or going to work out for a few minutes. But you did it and, assuming it was at least a little important to you, you managed to get it done.

2. *You (re)build confidence.* Cancer, at times, can kick your butt. Every once in a while, you need some type of personal victory to remind yourself that you are strong as a person and can actually get things done. Again, you don't have to go out and paint your house all alone or run a marathon. Small, smart, reasonable tasks in alignment with your physical and mental capabilities at the time will go a long way to helping you feel much less helpless.

3. *You have the opportunity to build momentum.* Let's say you get up early and make lunch for your kids one day. It wasn't terrible, and you could rearrange your sleep/nap schedule to account for it. Now, let's say you decide to do this for a few days in a row. Maybe you start on a Wednesday or Thursday and do it for two or three days. This is a case where everyone wins. You win because you decided to do something and built momentum. Your kids win because, even if only for a few days, you managed to return some small bit of normalcy to their lives. It's small, but it matters because it signals to them (and to you) that you are pushing to get things back to normal.

The obligatory caution I will give a million times is that y**ou have to listen to your body**. There is a fine line between wimping out of doing something you can and should do because you convince yourself that you aren't up to it and forcing yourself to do something you are not yet ready to do and paying the price. Newsflash, you aren't going to feel up to it for some time but make sure you know the difference.

The Important distinction is to be able to manage (in your head) the difference between being physically or mentally unable and *simply not wanting* to do something. Talk to your doctor, know your limits, get supervision if you have to, and then get going. Decide to do things, and then get them done. It's really the only way to make sure that you are PUSHING to get things back to normal. It's an active process that needs to start as quickly as possible once your treatment is completed and with the full participation of your medical team.

ON GETTING SUPERVISION

As you know or will find out, you can get pretty tired, pretty fast sometimes when you are in the middle of treatment. Sometimes, simply getting out of bed can be a challenge. What is important is that you think ahead and sort out whether you MAY need some help with whatever you are planning on doing.

Error on the side of caution when deciding if you need help.

For me, it was working out. We don't live in a neighborhood with sidewalks, so there wasn't any good place for me to walk around outside. It was also winter in Ohio (cold), so I didn't want to walk outside anyhow. My wife and I would go to our gym, and I would walk around the track some. She was always by my side, either literally (the first few workouts) or figuratively, working out so she could keep an eye on me. It's important while you are pushing yourself back to normalcy that you are smart about having a buddy help you when you think you could need it.

It's also 100% important to tell your doctor EXACTLY what you plan to do and get their permission or agreement. If your doctor says "no," then it's a "no."

Applied Determination—Shorter Chemo Cycle

My last round of chemo (which was by far the worst) was scheduled to end on a Saturday at around 3 PM. The problem with this schedule was that it was Senior Day for my oldest son, who was on the high school swim team. Normally, it wasn't an issue to show up late to a meet. But this was his last high school meet ever, and they had a whole big program where each swimmer's family was introduced with the swimmer in front of the whole natatorium. They receive flowers and announce where they are going to college—the whole nine yards.

The only problem for me was that I wasn't going to be able to make it. I was set to finish my chemo treatment too late. It also meant that unless my wife told me to take an Uber home from chemo, she wasn't going to make it either.

So, my goal was to get done early. I asked the doctor, and he said they could do the chemo routine in ninety hours instead of the usual ninety-six hours. This would get me done in time to stop home, change, and get to the pool on time. My doctor did some research and approved the shorter plan. He said that if the faster chemo rate was starting to cause additional challenges, they would put me back on the regular schedule. With a lot of research and hard work from my doctor, I was able to set my goal of getting to the meet in time to get introduced with my son.

After setting the goal, I worked hard to be a model patient for those ninety hours, knowing that I needed to be able to function and stay awake for a few hours past the time I was released. Then, I could go to bed and sleep. I ate (lots of homemade soup). I walked when I could, and, most importantly, I slept. I ended up tolerating the increased chemo drug rate OK but felt myself getting more tired each day and ended up getting a blood transfusion during this last chemo cycle. Finally, the morning of being released came. I felt pretty good in the morning, getting close to reaching my goal of getting out to the swim meet. I finished chemo and the cold bag and waited for discharge papers.

They spent about an hour getting my paperwork in order, and I started feeling dizzy. Not just a little dizzy but VERY dizzy. Those cold bags at the end of my chemo were the absolute worst for me. I sat for a bit and drank some Coke® (lots of fast sugar) and started feeling better. We came close to being tripped up, but we made it out right after getting my walking papers, and I was feeling OK. The rest of the day went as planned, and I made it to the meet on time, got home a few hours later, and had a VERY good sleep.

So what happened here? Let's think about it some:

1. I set a goal—a specific outcome with a date and time.
2. I got approval from my treatment team.
3. I figured out my part of the process.
4. I worked hard to deliver on my part of the process.
5. I got to celebrate a small success.

APPLIED DETERMINATION—HERE'S WHAT WORKED FOR ME

As I said, I am convinced that this concept can set your life back on a path where it can feel normal. At first, maybe only for a few moments, and then gradually, you can set yourself back on the path to a normal life.

Develop Your List of Goals, Both Big and Small

Start small and work yourself up. It can be anything. Some ideas are

- Make a batch of cookies or cook something.
- Do some activity with family or friends. Go to dinner. Take a walk.
- Go to the mall or grocery store.
- Do ten minutes on the elliptical machine or treadmill, or take a walk.
- Finish something for work.
- Write some thank you notes.

Decide When and Where

DO NOT, DO NOT, DO NOT skip this step. Give yourself a deadline. Otherwise, it's only a suggestion.

Plan Around the Goal

What possible physical (or mental) challenges will you have to manage to reach your goal?

Sign Off with Your Health Team

No, you are not running a marathon yet. Get permission or advice where needed. Figure out if you may need help or supervision from someone else—*i.e.*, exercise or diet changes.

Find Someone to Hold You Accountable or Help You

This could be family, friends, co-workers, or anyone who is enough of a pain in the butt to make sure you do it. Tell them what you are planning and, more importantly, WHY you are planning it.

Celebrate

Celebrate with a group hug or you lying in bed that night, congratulating yourself for a small win—whatever makes sense for you. *This is important.* So do it.

Plan the Next Goal

Momentum builds quickly with applied action.

A FINAL NOTE ON APPLIED DETERMINATION— MOVE YOUR BUTT

One of the things that was really helpful for me was moving. It didn't matter if I was taking laps around my chemo floor at the hospital (hospital staff got a real kick out of that), walking around in my house, or walking around the outside of my house. Movement helped me a lot. It wasn't always fun and didn't always feel great, but I did it. (My dirty little secret is that I didn't always want to do it, not by a mile.)

You will have a ready-made reason to be inactive. It's a good one too.

Don't use it.

Move your butt anyhow. Push yourself to do it. Assign someone to be your personal motivator. Motivate yourself, and move your butt. Walk the dog. Walk to the mailbox. Walk around your living room or even to the bathroom. Walk. Move, get vertical and get in motion.

What good comes of it?

It feels normal—even if only for a few minutes. You can actually forget you are sick sometimes.

It does help your body. It gets things moving, inside and out, and that's a good thing.

It provides a point of confidence. You did something positive and healthy.

Do it.

8

TREATMENT—DECIDED FAITH

Faith is taking the first step even when you
don't see the whole staircase.

—Martin Luther King, Jr.

Faith during your journey is important because, at some point, you will have to face the fact that cancer is pretty serious business and bad things can happen to you, including death. Your faith can be a large (and often primary) source of support as you go through the challenging portions of your treatment and recovery. It's important that you sort out what you think about things like life, death, heaven, prayer, and other faith concepts so you can rely on your faith for support through challenging times and encourage others to help you where appropriate. Whatever you believe, you will need that part of your life to be settled, or at least supportive, as you progress (and fight at times) through your treatment.

There is no wrong or right answer here, only the opportunity to leverage faith to help you through your cancer journey. You will decide, on purpose, to apply your faith in different ways to reduce the mental stress and doubts that almost always accompany a cancer diagnosis.

This, honestly, was the most challenging part of the book to think through and write. I don't think it is my place to tell anyone what to think about their own faith, so my advice is simply a practical approach to apply faith-based tools that provide support you during your cancer journey. They are based on a few simple observations or personal realizations. It's also important that you think about it some too. Faith is a vital part of your support system.

The goal of this chapter is twofold:

1. To share a few faith-based concepts that anyone can use as support when it is most needed.
2. To relate stories that cause you to think more about your faith and how you can apply it to lend support for your personal journey.

I think, at the most basic level, I settled on a few simple things where I used my faith or my understanding of my faith to support me during my cancer journey:

1. Your cancer is not some type of punishment by God.
2. Prayer is a powerful means of granting yourself some peace and is also a force multiplier.
3. You must decide, on purpose, to have faith that you will overcome your illness.

First, I will provide some background on myself from a faith perspective so you can at least understand where I am coming from.

MY FAITH BACKGROUND

I was raised "casually" Presbyterian. I say casually because we went to church every once in a while, maybe a few times a quarter, always at Christmas and Easter, along with a few stints in Vacation Bible School. It wasn't a perfect track record, but at least some semi-regular church. Now, this doesn't mean that I wasn't paying attention in church. I was paying attention, but I honestly didn't think too much about my faith until later in my life.

Fast forward to a few years after I was married. My wife is Catholic. Her family on both sides is Catholic—actually, very Catholic—to the point where her Uncle Ralph is a Catholic Priest. He married us. Once we had kids, I felt it was important that I convert to Catholicism so that we would have a consistent faith message for our kids. I had to go through the confirmation process as an adult. Weekly classes that touched on a wide variety of aspects of faith. It was interesting at times. Other times, it was pretty boring. When we were done, I was confirmed in the Catholic church. It was a big celebration at Easter. Everybody was happy.

What always struck me about pretty much anything in any church training is that they are telling you exactly what to think about different aspects of faith or religion. I understood the lessons, made my own interpretations, and actually got settled with my faith and its teachings long before I was sick—it was a huge source of strength. Not everyone is settled in their faith. For those cases, I will try to offer a way to look at things that works wherever you are on your journey to settling in your faith.

So, what does this mean regarding how you think about faith, and why does this matter when you are traveling through your cancer journey?

If you are fully settled in your faith, it makes it easier to use faith as a support to get you through the challenges of cancer. What exactly does it mean to be settled? There are a wide variety of theological definitions out there, but I will simplify it greatly for our purposes.

Being settled in your faith means you know what you believe in your heart and with unshakable conviction.

How you get to the point of being settled is probably another book that I am 100% unqualified to write. But think on it, read, study, pray, attend services, and keep doing these things until you have clarity in your mind regarding how YOU think faith works in your life.

THE HOSPITAL CHAPLAIN VISITS

My visits from the hospital chaplain are what helped me get my thoughts in some reasonable order on the subject of using faith as a means of support as a cancer patient.

When I was in the hospital for my first chemo round, I had a visit from the chaplain. She was very nice, had recently finished the balance of her formal schooling, and came to chat to see if I wanted to pray some and check in to see how I was doing.

Her questions, at the time, seemed off-target for where I was mentally. *Was I doing OK? Was I feeling stressed out? Did I experience anxiety? Was I scared? Was I feeling angry?* (At God is what she meant) Of course, I was feeling stressed out, but not in the way she was asking. It is stressful being in the hospital and being poked every two hours. No rest for the weary, as they say. That said, I didn't have the type of anxiety she appeared to be looking for. We said a prayer, and she went on her way, saying she would come back tomorrow or the next day.

No chaplain visited the next day. I guess I scared her off.

She came in the following day, and we started talking some more. She asked more of the same questions, but this time, she probed a bit more with the "tell me more about that" line of inquiry. Our conversations were always pretty helpful, so I answered the questions again, but this time with the "tell me more" additions.

It was a long discussion. As the chaplain asked questions, I asked about her experiences with people in my cancer hospital. Many were feeling angry at God. Many were feeling scared, and many were feeling overwhelmed (I'm hoping this book can help with that part). She had some great stories about how she was REALLY able to help people.

If you think about it, for a chaplain, it has to be a great gig. Captive, individual audiences, and many with a real spiritual need. It's different than preaching to the guy in a church of 500 people who is hoping that the homily ends fast so he can go home and mow his lawn before it rains.

When you are sick, you assume (for me, before thinking about it) that everyone responds to the challenges of diagnosis and treatment the same. When I experienced the fact that everyone's journey is VERY different by walking around a cancer floor for a few weeks, I started to ask why. At the most basic level, I settled on stress/overwhelm (lack of mental or other useful strategies) and different levels of faith.

SOME INSIGHTS PROMPTED BY THE CHAPLAIN

I've paraphrased some of the discussions I had with the chaplain, which were super helpful in clarifying my thoughts and providing me some peace as they occurred.

<u>On Being Angry</u>

Chaplain: "Are you angry?"

Me: "What for?"

Chaplain: "Some people get angry at the world or angry at God when they get very sick."

Me: "You are the expert, but I don't think God works like that."

Chaplin: "What do you mean?"

Me: "God doesn't give people cancer because they did something wrong."

Chaplain: "Yes, I think that's right."

<u>On Being Scared</u>

Chaplain: "Are you scared at all?"

Mc: "What do you mean?"

Chaplain: "Some people are scared of what could happen with their treatment."

Me: "Like what? It doesn't work?"

Chaplain: "Not exactly that."

Me: "I believe in heaven, and I will go there if I die. Is that what you mean?"

Chaplain: "No."

At this point, my guess is she felt as if the discussion was going off track. I was trained as a "cancer buddy" by my treatment hospital, and we were trained to stay away from these rabbit holes as it leads to negative thoughts and unproductive thinking. In general, it isn't in any way helpful.

Me: "I do not want to die. I am fighting like heck to do everything I can to be engaged with my treatment and to think and act in a way that is supportive of getting healthy again. But, if it's God's will, I will accept it."

I do need to elaborate here. This didn't mean I was OK with dying or that I had given up and thrown my recovery to the winds. What it meant was that I believe 100% in a higher power, and if I did everything I could to get healthy and it didn't work, and I passed, I believed I was going to heaven. That's being settled in your faith. It eliminates fear. It's kind of like the Bible passage about walking through the valley of death but not being scared.

From Psalm 23, King James Bible: Yea, though I walk through the valley of the shadow of death, I will fear no evil: for thou art with me; thy rod and thy staff they comfort me.

Look, the point here is that it helps to feel settled with your faith—wherever you are in your journey. Know what you believe 100% and then lean on it—hard. I was settled with my faith, and it helped me a lot. It can get pretty dark in your head at times. You feel worse than you have ever felt. You have more treatment ahead, no hair, and you can't manage your thoughts. So, it helps to have some sort of backstop. Faith is extra support for you. For me and for many people, it's the primary support.

When I thought about what to write about in this section, it came down to three things: punishment, prayer, and heaven. The chaplain's discussions prompted the punishment and heaven parts. The prayer part came later with a little different insight. I will elaborate in each of the sections and will even point out some things to help increase the probability that you are sorted with your faith if you aren't 100% there yet, at least to the point it is supportive of your treatment and recovery. If you are not 100% settled in your belief in these concepts, many times, with a little work and help from spiritual leaders, you can achieve it and realize more peace in the process.

The object here is to provide thoughts on using faith-based concepts to bring strength and comfort.

PART 1: PUNISHMENT—GOD DOES NOT PUNISH PEOPLE

When you are sick, you may try to find some reason that you got sick. I can tell you from experience it's not a particularly productive exercise. Four to five days inpatient for each chemo treatment, hopped up on steroids, and poked by nurses every two to four hours; there wasn't a lot of sleep. So, I had a lot of time to try to figure out how or why I got sick.

Even if you can point to things that may have helped cause your cancer, so what? You can't go backward, only forward. If you want to go down that road, focus on changing whatever behavior you think contributed to your cancer. In many cases, there won't be anything to point to, so let it go and focus 100% on getting better.

Often, patients can't point to what caused their cancer from the traditional list of typical physical causes. In these cases, you look elsewhere for explanations but don't have a lot of places to look, so you blame yourself. How? You think God is somehow punishing you with cancer for something you have done in your past. You can't come up with anything else, and since EVERYONE has done something they probably shouldn't have done, at least in the eyes of God, you are eligible to be punished.

The problem is that God doesn't work that way.

One of the two insights from my discussions with the Chaplain (and others) is the belief that God doesn't punish people—certainly not by giving them cancer. It's an important distinction that will bring you peace if you can get it settled in your head. The Chaplain mentioned the anger and guilt of a diagnosis are some of the main stressors for cancer patients outside of the fear of death. It's also clear that both of those stresses are entirely self-manufactured and completely unnecessary.

This simple realization that God or anyone else isn't punishing you can create peace for you on two levels *if you let it*:

1. You let go of the stress and guilt that comes with feeling like you somehow did something to "deserve" having cancer. It's simply

not the case. According to my psychologist friend, this is guilt, and it lets us know when we have done something to someone else who we may want to "fix."

2. You also get to let go of any anger you have about being sick. I don't have to tell you that being angry while also being sick isn't particularly helpful because you already know that. My psychologist friend tells me that anger is a means of protecting ourselves. He also says that research has shown that people who repress emotions may be more likely to develop cancer.

Someone explained it to me by likening God to a loving parent—disappointed when you do things wrong but always forgiving and not looking to dish out "punishment."

You are sick and not being punished by God, no matter your past. Believe it.

Part 2: Prayer—Prayer Matters

This is probably the most multi-faceted concept of the three concepts in this chapter. It is interesting because it's somewhat therapeutic (you ask for help), a source of support (others offer their prayers to you), and is the easiest point for many to cross over to being settled, at least in this one aspect of their faith.

To me, prayer is a means of asking for help. You admit that you need help and ask for it. It's pretty simple. I think for many people going through treatment, it's a natural response. You feel overwhelmed, uncertain, and stressed, so you reach out and ask for help. Most people won't ask for help publicly (this is why I am also 100% convinced that this book will be helpful to a LOT of people). If you pay attention, how often you pray can also gauge how stressed/overwhelmed/anxious you are feeling. Reaching out with specific requests is a recognition that you want help. Depending on your headspace, you will be asking for needed additional help or asking for help as another action on your part to do everything possible to get better.

Take some quiet time to pray for strength, health, recovery, sanity, or whatever else you need.

There have been myriad studies on prayer (and intention), and all of them seem to point to the benefit of prayer and intention having some ability to influence outcomes.

Let Others Pray For You

Prayer is also a prime opportunity to ask others for help or direct them to an easy but very meaningful way to help you.

Honestly, I didn't learn this until a few years after I was done with my adventure. I was hanging out with a fraternity brother I hadn't seen in years, and he found out through my son about my lymphoma. He asked me, rather pointedly, why I never told him. I shot back, "What were you going to do?" He said he would have prayed for me.

This was a huge light bulb moment for me.

One of the things you will recognize pretty quickly is that you will have a bunch of random people wanting to help you. When I say random, it's not COMPLETELY random, as in some guy picked your name from the phone book. More likely, especially in supportive communities, it will be someone you have met and been cordial with who genuinely wants to find a way to support you. It's an old friend, or you coached their kid in sports, or you go to the same church, etc.

When they ask what they can do, ask them to pray for you. I 100% believe that prayer helps in many ways. It's one leg in your faith support system. After reflection, I sorted out that asking others to pray for you is a high leverage but still private way to have people you don't know very well to provide some level of support.

I have a grand total of one easy-to-comprehend prayer example that illustrates how prayer works, at least in my mind.

Prayer Before Milling

We recently had a guy over to our house to mill some trees we had cut down into lumber. He is a good Christian man and asked if we could pray before he started working. We said fine. (I hadn't ever prayed with anyone who came to help at my house, but I was fine with it.) We prayed for a good day, good yields, safety, and a good experience for everyone with no problems. *Good plan*, I thought to myself.

Late in the day, there was a big problem. His sawmill lost a bolt with a lock nut (if you don't know what that is, it really doesn't matter to the story). We couldn't find it in the now huge pile of sawdust. We looked with our hands and a metal detector but had no luck. It was gone. He couldn't work anymore without replacing the bolt.

I told him I would run down to my basement and see if I had anything that could work. He needed an industrial size bolt and a locking nut. I guessed no way I would have what we needed. For the layperson, pretty much all of the nuts and bolts I have are the thickness of a chopstick. He needed something as thick as your pinky finger and a locking nut to boot. No way would I have that, but I figured I would at least look.

I looked through all of my jars of spare nuts and bolts—probably a thousand or more. They were all pretty small (chopstick size). I got to the last jar, and when I turned it over, I saw something that looked huge—it was way bigger than any other bolt I had, and it had a lock nut. I took it outside to see if the size and threading were close so we could use it temporarily. We tried the bolt in the hole, and it's the EXACT size he needed: the right threading, the right length, and a lock nut.

If you told me you would give me a million dollars to explain where it came from, I would still have no idea. I'm not implying that it appeared as if by magic but simply relating that I never have any call to use industrial-size bolts in my everyday "handyman" duties.

You make your own decision on how this happened, but, as I said, I had never prayed with anyone who came to help at my house before this day, and this whole situation seemed to work out way too perfectly.

PART 3: FAITH SUPPORT AND DECIDED FAITH

Leveraging Religious Faith as Support

Everyone is at a different place regarding how well they are settled with their religious faith. When you are sick, it can be a time for reflection, accelerated learning, and personal growth. It's probably not the right time to add the stress to your life to "figure out" or settle your foundational faith beliefs if they aren't already in place.

No matter where you are on your faith journey, you can get at least some support from your religious faith. Aside from praying, you can focus and meditate on the support you receive from your personal "higher power." For me, being fully settled in my religious faith gave me the ability to "let go" at times of extreme fear, worry, or stress. I think that no matter where you are on your religious faith journey, use that faith to aid in simply letting go and trusting in a higher power.

Faith Another Way—Have Faith in the Process

As you go through treatment, sometimes it's hard to believe you are on track to recovery. Some crazy things can happen with your treatment, the recovery process, and side effects, among other things. As these things happen, you start coming back to the feelings of fear, worry, and stress associated with not knowing exactly what happens next and how long your personal process may take. It's merely another distraction that has the potential to get you off track.

In addition to working through some of the other strategies offered here, I have one other (non-religious) faith suggestion to offer.

Decide, on purpose, to have faith that you will recover from your illness.

Again, it's a choice. It's a way of thinking. It's another means of fighting off the negative things that come with expected or unexpected stress.

For me, it was tough to adhere to at times.

Here is another perspective shared with me by Rita Alarcon, a fellow cancer survivor and author of *Leave Me Breastless—A Journey of Grace, Listening and Trust*:

> "In prayer and faith in life and life's processes, it is not that we will not encounter problems, but rather a trust that we are supported in the challenges we face and that those challenges may mold us into the person we are meant to be."

9

POST TREATMENT—BE FEARLESS

You woke up today. Might as well be a badass.
—Robin Arzon, Peloton Instructor

My brother-in-law reminds me that there is always a doctor's appointment on the schedule for me and every other cancer patient and survivor unless you have been out of the tank (hospital) for a very long time—usually five years or more. This is true. I always have another appointment on the schedule, and as I write this, I am on a six-month schedule with the doctor. Bloodwork, checkups, and visit with the doctor each time. They ask how I feel, if I fell, and if there is anything noteworthy going on with my health, at least anything noteworthy that doesn't show up in their charts.

The first few appointments—scheduled monthly—were easy. It seemed like a logical continuation of my treatment. They weren't scary; it felt like more of the same as when I was in the tank. When the appointments moved to every three months, it started to get a little interesting, at least in my head, until I put a stop to it. It's another iteration of having to manage your headspace.

I thought when I was done, I was done, but the reality was that I was pretty sick. It sucked, to be sure, and it could have caused me to die. As I said before, that's pretty serious stuff. Given all of this recent experience, your bias is to not want your cancer to return and a fear it might. I fell into the fear trap until I thought about it purposefully.

As anyone who lives and breathes, you know your body doesn't work like a robot. You sleep on your neck funny, and it hurts; you chase the dog too long, and maybe your legs are sore. You go to spinning class and go really hard for thirty minutes, and you feel it the next day. Or maybe you simply sit up too fast and get dizzy. There are always some SMALL things going on in your body as it works with you to adjust to everyday life.

To someone who never had cancer, these minor physical ailments are only something you deal with—another physical bump on the road of life but nothing to worry about. Not noteworthy. To a cancer survivor, it usually commands more attention. The evaluation moves to whether or not the current physical difficulty somehow indicates you're sick again.

I honestly let my head go there for a short period after I progressed to check-up appointments that were three or six months apart. Then, I thought about it critically: over a few beers, in the shower, on a late-night plane flight—I'm not sure where and when exactly I sorted this in my mind. I was so tired I didn't have the energy to worry; there was only enough energy to work through more functional solutions to my worry.

- Did I have any reason to believe that the three or six-month interval for checkups was too short?
- Was I withholding information from the doctors that might indicate some issue or warrant further medical investigation?
- Did I feel that I was being honest with myself about minor physical issues I felt between appointments? Did I underestimate these issues or discount them?
- And finally, the most important question—what could I accomplish by worrying?

As you work out your approach to how to handle this, here are a few things to think about:

1. It is very likely that the things that were done to your body to heal it of cancer were also highly abusive. Some of the abuse done to your body takes time to heal or get sorted. Ask anyone who has had very intensive chemo or radiation treatment.

2. If you start pushing yourself physically after treatment (I am assuming your doctor agrees with this), you will experience some pain or discomfort as you try to push yourself back to the level of physical health you desire. Listen to your body and stop when you need to but don't use it as an excuse.

3. Explain exactly what you are doing (or planning on doing) with your doctor on your checkup visits. Are you fasting? Are you doing some type of diet, or are you training for a marathon? Give them a chance to evaluate what you are doing or planning on doing to avoid issues ahead of time.

You will likely have a lot of mental (am I still OK?) and physical (does that pain in my leg mean something?) challenges starting right after you finish treatment. What is the best way, in my estimation, to handle them?

Be fearless.

Live your life. Reach for your goals. Go get it. Say whatever you say to yourself to indicate that you are back and doing what YOU want to do when you want to do it.

When you break down the two areas you may struggle with post-treatment—mental and physical—it becomes easy to rationalize your worries away.

On the mental side, whatever you have made up as a concern is more than likely "made up"—if you had real issues, your doctor would tell you. This doesn't mean that if you are struggling with a mental health crisis, you should forget about it or try to ignore it. In that case, raise your hand and ask for help—now.

For the garden variety things you make up to worry about, find something else to focus on. Cancer doesn't define you; if it's over, it's over—get on with your life. Even better, use the experience as a point of reflection and sort out how you choose to approach life going forward.

You were given an invaluable life lesson—use it!

On the physical side, you will have some pain or discomfort popping up in different places in your body, especially if you are older. It's called being old. Set up your physical goals (workouts, diet, etc.), get approval from your doctor, and start moving. Go do your thing. Work hard, focus, and regain your physical health. Catalog whatever discomfort you feel, talk through it at your checkups, and decide with your doctor if there is some concern.

Be Fearless—Here's What Worked for Me

On being mentally fearless:

1. This is another "get yourself together" moment. Again, you are in the position of having to notice and then take active control of your thoughts. Take some time to get clarity on the fears exposed as you "worry" about the future and your cancer.

2. Listen to your self-talk and make adjustments where necessary. The strategies are the same ones we discussed in Chapter 3: Get Yourself Together. As you recognize worries, make sure to append or replace the thoughts with something more positive.

3. Make the transition away from living in fear and the past. Your cancer is done. It's over. Act that way. Sometimes, it takes a bit to get back to a normal routine. Take the opportunity to create an "improved" new normal. Eat better, exercise more, meditate—whatever resonates with you. Leverage the fact that you were sick to appreciate the opportunity to simply live your life every single day after your recovery.

4. Do things on purpose that are physically demanding and a little scary; it flexes both your mental and physical muscles. Run a race, take a course, go on a travel adventure; you get the picture. Take the opportunity to build mental confidence.

On being physically fearless:

1. Pay attention to how you feel physically. There is a fine line between simply being aware and being over-attentive to every little thing that bothers you. Sore muscles, aches, occasional headaches, and occasional bouts of an upset stomach become part of everyday life. Be honest but fair with yourself. Let minor physical difficulties go for a few days to see if they resolve themselves. If not, tell your doctor. Call right away on things that are serious.

2. If you are physically well, look for opportunities to prove it to yourself. Be smart about how you push, but push yourself physically, at least a little, to improve your health and mental toughness. It also provides a recent point of reference that supports the fact that your physical health has been restored. Run, ride, walk, swim, or do whatever you do to build your physical strength.

3. Allow yourself to dwell on your physical success. This flexes your mental muscles while leaning on a reference point for some type of physical success. Think about a physical achievement, even a small one, every day until you create another physical success. I remember the day that I was finally able to achieve my pre-cancer output on an elliptical machine. It was ugly, but I did it and proved, at least to myself, that my physical health was on the mend.

Be fearless.

10

HOW TO HELP AS AN ADVOCATE

Service to others is the rent you pay for your room here on earth.

—Mohammed Ali

I n Chapter 4: Advocate for Yourself, we talked about the absolute 100% need to advocate for yourself throughout your diagnosis, treatment, and recovery. We also said that if you couldn't or wouldn't advocate for yourself that you should find someone to do it for you. This chapter is directed toward the person you've chosen to advocate for you.

To the appointed advocate—

Being an advocate for someone who is sick is one of the most important roles you can perform for them. Take the responsibility seriously. It matters—a lot. You also have to plan to be present (in person) for all important conversations.

One other note is that there can only be one "lead" advocate. Let the patient make the call and go from there.

What Advocacy Means—Your Responsibilities

Your role as an advocate is to

1. Fully UNDERSTAND where your patient is in the process and what is coming, at least a few weeks in advance. This means that you not only understand what is happening in the next few hours and days, but it means you have done your homework to understand the planned treatment process as far out as possible. It also means that if something sneaks up on you (unexpected or unknown treatment), you ask if it will be a regular or one-time item. In my experience, many procedures are ordered "just in time." Sometimes these things happen, but, at the same time, there are often patterns. You also need to understand what is going on in the patient's everyday personal life because it doesn't simply stop for them while they are in treatment.

2. HELP your patient manage the decision process for the optional parts of the treatment. Sometimes there is some flexibility in parts of treatment (for example, whether a procedure is done, a shot is given, or the timing of a particular part of treatment). Your job is to help your patient walk through the pros and cons of each option WITH their care team and arrive at a choice that makes sense for them. You are objective when helping sort these decisions simply by helping review the pros and cons of each side of these optional treatments.

3. FIND areas of treatment flexibility that would be helpful or more comfortable for the patient. This means asking a lot of questions to see whether there are options concerning the timing or intensity of different parts of treatment or protocols that you know would be of huge benefit to your patient. Some examples might be the timing of treatment to allow for more sleep or diet flexibility to allow for more homemade food or excursions outside the hospital to get some fresh air or gain a different perspective. All of this is done with the full knowledge and consent of the treatment team. Be respectful and reasonable in your requests, and the care team will always reciprocate if they can. Take a "no"

as a "no." Healthcare professionals aren't saying "no" to these types of requests to be difficult.

4. Fully COMMUNICATE whatever you find out with the patient. The timing of when you tell the patient good or bad news is up to you, but nothing short of full disclosure is appropriate.

5. TELL the doctor everything you know about the patient that concerns their physical or mental health. If you need to talk privately with the doctor or nurse about the patient, then do it.

I will make this point again: *You are not a doctor or a medical professional. Do what they say.* Know your role.

Ask a ton of questions, understand the treatment process, and find areas of possible flexibility with the treatment process, then do what you can to implement things that make the process smoother and less stressful for the patient.

WHAT A PATIENT NEEDS

Patients need less stress. If you understand the stressors affecting the patient and what you can do to help reduce them, you can be effective as an advocate. Most of the stress experienced by a cancer patient is caused by one of three things:

1. Fear of the unknown or unknowable

2. Feeling uncomfortable—mentally or physically

3. Feeling overwhelmed to some degree

If you can work a little bit in these three areas, you should be able to help reduce the stress levels and help your patient get the best possible treatment outcome with the least possible stress.

FEAR OF THE UNKNOWN—HOW YOU CAN HELP

This section is an information-gathering exercise (yes, go buy a notebook—see below). When you come forward as an advocate, your goal should be to get ahead of what is coming toward your patient. Initially, you will have to understand the present situation and what is coming next.

Find out who is who. That means you know which care provider is responsible for every test or procedure being contemplated and who is in charge of different portions of the care currently being received. As you will find out, your patient will have several different caregivers throughout their treatment. Find out who does what, how to contact them, and what situations should prompt a call. This is also a huge opportunity to get inside information by building real relationships with the care team to get their professional insight as someone who helps patients manage their daily cancer treatment process. They have more experience. Do your best to tap into it. Don't monopolize their time—do be ready with good questions when you have the chance to ask.

Fear of the Unknown—Here's What Worked for Me

1. Understanding the process as far into the future as you can is the most important task. Also, explicitly ask what complications or negative outcomes are possible with each treatment or procedure. Start outlining how you might help your patient deal with these outcomes should they occur.

2. Gather the names and contact numbers (and emergency numbers) of all caregivers, the hospital, clinic, pharmacy, mental health professionals, etc. Know how to contact everyone you might have to on behalf of your patient.

3. Find who, what, and when for different situations that could arise. Who do you call, under what conditions, and when is it an emergency or the time to call? One example might be if your patient is in chemo and has a fever for longer than two hours; you may have to call your patient's doctor or go to the ER. (This isn't medical advice; it's only an example.). It's about thinking ahead.

4. Ask the treatment team questions that are important to your patient. You need to do some homework to see what your patient is interested in learning. You likely know them very well, so you should be able to gather information relevant to your patient. Some examples might be when the patient will be cleared for exercise again or how whether certain diet choices are advisable with the current treatment. After you have a clear understanding of the treatment plan—move to the "lifestyle" questions that are sure to arise.

The Notebook

I previously mentioned that you need a notebook. Yes, pen and paper (at least for now). Why? So both you and your patient can write in it, and the information in it can be shared but, most importantly, recorded. You need a notebook with a calendar and it has to be a large enough area to record daily events and add other information, such as questions, complications, etc.

So, what goes in the notebook, exactly? Whatever you want to put in it, but, at a minimum, I would include the following four things:

The Big Picture Calendar—Getting Out Front

In your notebook, write down hour by hour, day by day, or week by week, the exact list of planned procedures. During doctor visits, try to push out your understanding of the schedule as far as possible. For example, let's say there are three weeks of chemo left on a regular schedule. Make sure you start asking now exactly what happens next. Now, do the same thing for your patient's personal schedule: family events, work commitments, travel schedules, etc.

Note What You Learned

Take careful notes, and don't feel bad asking for things to be repeated. Doctors, nurses, and other caregivers are busy people, so don't belabor points if it's not necessary. Take notes on procedures and record all the possible complications and recommendations the doctors give.

Contact Information for Treatment Team Members

Write down the contact information for every caregiver and resource you can. Make sure you know who to call and when.

Write Down Questions

Have the notebook handy at all times—you will forget to ask a lot of the questions you had that weren't written down. It's the most efficient approach for you, your patient, and the care team. Your care team won't have to patiently wait for you to remember (or search for) questions.

BEING UNCOMFORTABLE—HOW YOU CAN HELP

Cancer is pretty awful—that is a fact. Sometimes, the worst part is the discomfort caused by aspects of the treatment process: aches, pain, treatment scars, plus all the things that treatment can do to mess up your insides. The treatment team is always the place to start with these discomforts to see where medical intervention may help.

There are, however, a few different places where, as an advocate, you can significantly reduce or help accommodate the discomfort your patient feels in the treatment process. It can take many forms, and it's not always directly related to physical discomfort. An easy place to offer assistance is to ease their discomfort with how daily household items are handled (oftentimes by others) while a patient is in treatment.

It comes down to medically and non-medically addressable discomfort. We will talk about both.

Medically Addressable Discomfort

The treatment team likely knows whether and when a patient may encounter some discomfort. They are usually ready with some type of intervention that can be helpful. This usually takes the form of some kind of medicine to reduce pain, constipation, headache, and the like. Your job in this area is twofold:

1. Learn what options and process flexibility are available. Take every occasion to sort this ahead of time. For instance, if your patient is having a procedure and pain is listed as a side effect or a possible complication, find out at that time what pain management options may be available and how they can be deployed.

2. Help your patient inform the treatment team when a medical intervention for some type of discomfort is not working and ask for alternatives. Keep pressing the treatment team for more effective options if the current course of treatment isn't working. You should know that sometimes, there isn't a better or more effective alternative.

ONLY employ medical professional-approved medical intervention. This isn't the time to get creative.

Non-Medically Addressable Discomfort

Everything else that isn't treated or handled by a medical professional falls into this bucket. Some people complain 24/7, and in those cases, it's easy to try to find things to work on for your patient. Other patients are more subtle in communicating their discomfort, so you really have to pay attention. I will give three examples that outline how this can work for a patient so you have a place to start.

1. Food—Unless they have been living on the space station for a year, your patient hates hospital food. Even if they aren't spending time in the hospital, there is a strong likelihood that food simply tastes different than it used to for your patient. Sometimes, a patient needs a very strict diet; other times, not so much. Find out exactly where the boundaries are with food and diet for your patient. If they are in chemo, things will taste different, so you need to find maximum diet flexibility and take advantage. It was a breakthrough when I was allowed to have food, specifically soup, brought in for me, stored in the hospital refrigerator, and heated up when I was hungry. It was unbelievable how great that was. Some foods that may be helpful with side effects may be concerning to the care team. For example, some of my care team was very concerned with taking probiotics, so do your best to be specific with questions. Also, if your patient is experiencing a metallic taste in their mouth, they may be able to eat with plastic cutlery to reduce the effect.

2. Sleep—Sleep was always tough to come by for me, especially in the hospital with the checkups every few hours. The nurses would change the morning blood draw times to coincide with the blood pressure and other checkups so I could sleep longer, but it wasn't initially helpful because of the stupid monitor in the hospital computer in my room. My wife and I later kept asking the nurses how to turn the monitor off (it was super bright, especially at night). No one knew how to do it. So, my wife and I kept pushing and joking about how no one knew how to do it until a nurse manager finally got with the IT people to get some instructions printed.

   When dealing with a treatment regime in a home setting, make sure you do what you can to help clear the patient's schedule and create a very quiet and dark space to rest, anytime, day or night.

3. Move—If your patient is able, go for a walk with them or do some other approved physical activity to get them moving.

4. Distract—Change the focus to something else for your patient. Call a mutual friend or family member. Watch an inspirational

movie. Listen to music. Play cards. Do anything you can to distract from the discomfort intentionally.

OVERWHELM—HOW YOU CAN HELP

It's pretty easy to feel overwhelmed as a cancer patient, especially if your patient has a very invasive treatment regime, as I experienced. As we all know, "regular" life keeps going on: kids, parents, jobs, kids, dogs, bills, weather, etc. It all keeps rolling ahead on the day-to-day schedule, exactly as before your patient got sick. Add in the inability to physically or mentally complete or respond to some of these everyday items, and you can see how overwhelm can affect your patient.

Your job as an advocate is threefold in this area:

1. As you get out front in your understanding of the treatment process so you can help your patient, you do the same thing with their day-to-day, non-medical challenges or schedule to the extent needed or practical. What is the TOTAL picture, and are you helping your patient stay ahead of avoidable stress or issues? This means that you employ a combination of schedule simplification and adding additional resources to help complete some tasks where possible.

2. You run interference to block or reduce the impact of things you know will cause additional stress for your patient.

3. You call on additional resources where needed: more home support, mental health help, more community support, working with social workers, whatever is needed to round out the team advocating for your patient and preventing or addressing overwhelm.

Overwhelm—Here's What Worked for Me

<u>Clear the Plate</u>

Do everything you can to reduce the number of things that the patient must address from a non-medical perspective. This includes both personal and treatment-related items. Some examples might be cooking meals for the patient's family, getting the mail, picking up a prescription, letting nurses know preferences with respect to visitors, being attentive to desired room or home temperature, etc. Identifying and doing these tasks for your patient is the single biggest point of leverage in helping them reduce overwhelm.

<u>One Day (or One Hour) at a Time</u>

When your patient comes to the point of overwhelm, it can be helpful to reduce the time frame of focus to something manageable. When I started treatment, the list of procedures and possible complications was inordinately long and stretched over several months. Break it down for your patient. The "first" anything (procedure, chemo treatment, complication, radiation, etc.) is usually a good time to be on high alert because that is typically the time of maximum information flow to the patient. There is a huge opportunity to "slow things down" for your patient if you simply focus on shorter periods of time.

<u>Call For Help</u>

If your patient needs some outside help mentally processing their treatment experience or stress, then ask for it early. If you aren't sure whether your patient needs help, ask for it. It's way better to be early or overly cautious on this point rather than late. If you aren't comfortable asking for this resource for your patient, step aside for someone who is. It's that important.

A Final Note to Advocates and Caregivers

<u>Put on Your Own Oxygen Mask First</u>

The role of the caregiver is a serious role. It can take an emotional and physical toll on the caregiver. Know when you need a break, even a five-minute walk, or sitting in nature. If you need to call in a backup to refill your energy, do it. Lean into your patient's perspective, but keep boundaries for both of your sakes.

11

GENERAL POINTERS

Social media are junk food for our brains.

—Jonathan Salen Baskin, *Forbes Magazine*

Here are some things I found helpful during my treatment and why I decided to add these rules to my personal experience. Before I get started, I want to reiterate that if you feel for some reason that you want to harm yourself or feel hopeless, reach out and get professional help right away. There are ALWAYS resources—ask.

Now on to the general pointers.

STAY OFF SOCIAL MEDIA WITH YOUR STORY. PUT YOURSELF IN LOCKDOWN

Not everyone will agree with this, but here is my reasoning. Your diagnosis is personal; it's a personal fight, no matter how many people you have surrounding and supporting you. They don't feel what you feel and don't have the same fears and mental challenges. They are not in it. Many people won't or can't understand what you are going through and probably don't know what to say.

Social media is a bit of a disaster as I write this. Your story and plight are likely to be spread far and wide once you start posting it on social media, regardless of your alleged privacy settings. It can create issues, upset, and, most importantly, a loss of focus. You will likely have some people reaching out that you don't know very well. I suspect they will mean well, but it can be awkward and must be managed once it starts. There are a million other "not positive" outcomes from posting on social media. You can figure them out yourself.

Put yourself in lockdown. Choose, on purpose, who you share your story with, how you share it, and when you share it. Do it personally, on the phone, or via email. If someone reaches out to you, choose how to engage them. If you don't want to deal with someone who reached out, have one of your advocates deal with them for you. If you want to engage, do it on your schedule and terms.

Look, you have a lot going on and need 100% of your time and attention available to evaluate and generate helpful thinking around your diagnosis and treatment. Take time for yourself FIRST. Once you are squared away in your mind, THEN let others in. The only exception is cases where you know you need professional help. If that's the case, drop everything and make the call for help right away.

Answer this question: How many of your old friends would take your call your call out of the blue to tell them you have cancer and need to talk? My guess is it's close to 100%. Don't give up the opportunity to *choose* the people you engage with as you go through the process. Some people are WAY more helpful than others; determine the people who are helpful and have them help you. The easiest way to do this is to go into lockdown.

Your close friends and family (your people) will be there for you 100%, whatever the case.

QUEUE UP THE FUNNY STUFF

Laughter is an important part of getting through difficult treatments. Pretty much everyone has access to a phone and an internet connection nowadays. Think of things that make you laugh, find them on YouTube, and watch them—a lot. Doing this is a huge win from a few perspectives:

1. It passes the time. Sometimes, you really need to pass the time. Remember my suggestion of learning patience?

2. It changes your outlook. There are many scientific studies on laughter, and it works to help keep or get you healthy. If you read my blogs, you know I spent a lot of time trying to find humor in my adventures. It helped me get through, and even better, it helped me to laugh.

HARDEN YOUR BODY BEFORE YOU START TREATMENT—IF YOU CAN

Step one is to ask your doctor. If they say it's OK, go and do it.

If you have the chance and your doctor agrees, make sure you exercise, eat right, and get a bunch of sleep between the time of your diagnosis and when your treatment begins (and even during treatments). You will have a lot going on but prioritize this every day. Exercise as much as you can be based on any limitations you have or what your doctor tells you.

Your body is going to be abused somehow in order to eliminate your cancer. You will be irradiated, poisoned, and maybe even cut on—or worse. Toughen up ahead of time and while you can during treatment. Even if it's a few good workouts and a few strong, healthy meals before you start treatment, do it. It will help, at least a little bit.

I missed out on the ability to "get ready" due to my leg surgeries. I honestly think it put me a little behind the curve when I started chemo because my surgical wounds were still healing, and I couldn't exercise until well into my first chemo round.

EAT BETTER BUT AT LEAST EAT SOMETHING

I don't have to explain this one. You know the drill: fewer processed foods and more lean meats, fruits, veggies, and the like. Give your body a chance before and during treatment by not forcing it to deal with crappy food. Considering the abuse your body will be taking and all of the medicines your body and liver will be processing, at least give it a chance to repair itself quickly by providing the building blocks for repair through proper nutrition. If you don't know what that is exactly, ask for help. Every hospital or care center has or has access to a nutrition staff.

For me, it was soup, Gatorade®, protein drinks, cookies, and ice cream. I know I just gave you the lecture on eating well, and no, I wasn't eating equal parts soup, ice cream, and cookies. I ate mostly soup, but when I was feeling really bad, I included some protein drinks and ice cream. The protein drinks got me some decent nutrition, and the ice cream added calories and energy and soothed my mouth sores.

I will sum it up like this: eat healthy fuel for your body when you can, but when you are really out of sorts and can barely bring yourself to eat, eat something—anything—to get some nutrition and calories in you. I took this approach from some of my oncology nurses, who were thrilled to give me only Coke for eight hours when I was really, really worn out and didn't want to eat. Over and over, they said, "At least it's something to get some calories in you."

As always, talk with your doctor about this. I am merely relating what worked for me.

I have some soup and cookie recipes and some great places to get ice cream listed at the end of the chapter.

No Politics

I suppose it is not a revelation that the politics in most countries are becoming more polarized by the day. Each side has certain proof that the other side is awful for some reason or the other.

There are a lot of people who are paid a lot of money to get you riled up about the other side so you keep coming back to watch or read more to find out when the other side is FINALLY going to get what's coming to them. I will give you the answer now; it's never. They will never get the bad guys on the other side. Stay away from this nonsense and edit it from your life, at least while you are sick.

There is always something to learn about through reading or watching something on TV or online. Find it and turn off the politics.

DESIGNATE YOUR LAUGHTER PERSON

Everyone has someone they laugh with: a friend, spouse, a co-worker. There is always someone. Tell that person you need them on standby and ask them to make you laugh when you really need it. Have them on standby—really.

ANIMALS

This one almost got a whole chapter in the book. I suppose I should lay out what I believe with respect to animals (in this case, mostly dogs and cats) and how they read and respond to you.

I think that dogs (especially) and cats can sense exactly how you are from a mood and vitality standpoint, and they can use that information to respond to exactly how you are feeling and give appropriate support where needed. In short, they know when you are sick. I think it's something learned over many generations; they somehow know instinctively. I will leave it up to the professionals to sort out how.

I think it's a huge opportunity for you if you own a pet. It's another leg in your support system. It's another resource, another friend, and another opportunity to talk to a sympathetic listener.

We had recently gotten a puppy when I started treatment. Piper, a Fox Red Labrador Retriever, was the runt of the litter and about eight weeks old when we got her. We picked her up a few weeks before I first saw the doctor for my tumor. By the time I started treatment, she was several months old and very active. She was a typical puppy: jumping on everyone, wanting to be outside all the time, and constantly wanting to play.

Fast forward to chemo. My chemo cycles were four days, typically starting on a Monday, every three weeks. The low point of each cycle was about ten days after I started each cycle. The low was typically me laying on the couch 10+ hours a day for a few days when I was not in bed sleeping. I gradually got better from there during each cycle.

Piper, still a puppy, seemed to be able to sense how she should react to whatever my condition was at the moment. When I was at the lowest point of a treatment cycle, she would lay next to me for long periods, which was very unnatural for a puppy (or even a full-grown lab). When I was near the end of the cycle and feeling better, she would lobby to go outside more by scratching at the door or jumping up and lying in my lap. She knew I could, so she resumed lobbying to play or go outside. She was encouraging me to move my butt.

So, don't get a puppy or kitten if you are already sick, but if you have a dog or a cat, rely on the fact that they can sometimes know exactly how to be helpful and engage them in the process. It can be invaluable, especially in the middle of the night when everyone else is sleeping.

Practical Advice—No Gobbledygook

The internet is a dangerous place for a cancer patient. You will find a lot of information—oftentimes conflicting—about your diagnosis, type of cancer, your treatment, etc. You have to be very careful with researching on the web or using it as a resource when you are a patient.

When you are in or entering treatment, you need to get into a mental flow, a process. This means that you understand your diagnosis, treatment, and the path forward. It also means that you have a STABLE foundation from which to build out your response and the actions that will help you recover. Researching on the web will almost always result in uncovering differing opinions on one or more of your fundamental understandings of your situation. If you read all of the different opinions and take them as an authority, you will never get fully settled in your foundational beliefs about your situation.

This is why it helps to develop the skill of Studied Indifference. You have to study your situation and what your doctor is telling you and fully understand it from beginning to end. Ask all of your questions at the onset of your diagnosis. Process the information, build your foundational understanding of YOUR situation, then start to focus on treatment. Don't go back and begin to question your diagnosis, treatment, etc., by doing your own research each day. Develop your plan for your diagnosis with your doctor and stick to it.

There is one VERY glaring exception to this rule: you may need to rethink your situation with your doctor (or another doctor) if you aren't making progress. This is a sticky situation, but you need to evaluate whether the path you have traveled in a treatment program fits one of the possibilities laid out for you at the onset of treatment. If the results you are seeing are inconsistent with the list of possible outcomes or if your doctor seems flummoxed, it's probably time to reevaluate the situation and think about a second opinion.

THE HOSPITAL BAG

If you have to go inpatient for anything, spend a few minutes thinking ahead about what to bring with you. Here is a good list that was recommended to me:

- Notebook, pen/pencil
- Toothbrush, toothpaste, face and shower soaps
- Warm fuzzy socks, a soft pillowcase, an extra blanket (aka a woobie in our house), eyeshades, and earplugs
- Smartphone, iPad, headphones, books, magazines
- Lemon or ginger drops for nausea
- Plastic cutlery
- Emergency contact numbers, doctor numbers, insurance cards, living will, and other possible needed legal documents

BONUS: MY CANCER BLOGS

MONDAY—DAY 1 ROUND 1

Called hospital on way back from Starbucks at 8:00 am, bed is ready—Room 1630—they say come on down. Good start. I am happy. Arrive a check in, lady checking me in has very short hair, strange hair but she seems very nice. Getting checked in and I notice a lot of burns on her chest—I didn't ask why—that would be a bit creepy. She checks me in—got almost done getting checked in but something in the system is jacked up and I can't get 100% checked in. She calls guy in from across the hall to help, he says hit F7 to fix issue—but the F7 key—she no workee. They start a chat with IT and kick me out and say they will get me in a moment. Go out to lobby to wait. I go to take a pee and get a free candy cane on the way back for some reason- "Happy Holidays" I am told. Julie happy to get free candy upon my return. We wait for two minutes and the registration lady comes out to take us to our room. Success.

On the way to the room, the registration lady comments about the burns on her neck—they are from radiation. She is recently back from being out for several months and had some cancer I never heard of. She was super nice and positive.

Arrive at room 1630. Room is very nice and clean. Very nice view of Ohio Stadium, the towers, and other campus buildings. Room is private, which is good. I set down my belongings and the nurse shows up. We make some small talk—she is hoping I can start chemo

TODAY, by the end of the day. This, of course is a bit of a shock. I withhold the urge to say WTF. I was under the impression that I was starting right away—this is not the case. This is the beginning of unraveling the sandbagging of communication the full series of steps to get started with the chemo treatment. Not pleased. Doing the math now—I will get out mid-day on Saturday if I start tomorrow.

Helicopter flying towards my window now—looks ominous. Closer, closer then swerves at the last minute to land on helipad, which, by my count is about 100 feet as the crow (or helicopter) flies from my room. Not super loud. Expect lots of helicopters now 24/7— these fears later proven to be unfounded. Guessing that Friday will be a big helicopter day.

Back to nurse, she is looking for a vein to start an IV. Spends a long time surveying both arms and finds one she likes. I appreciate this approach as it improves chances of getting it right in one shot. Student nurse also here. She is apparently about done with schooling enough to take the boards but is taking another year and a half of schooling to get certified as a psych nurse. Student and regular nurse going over the finer points of putting in an IV and student nurse makes comment that actual practice is rarely like it is taught in class. Regular nurse and I get a big laugh out of this. Tourniquet only to be applied for a set # of seconds according to student—totally unrealistic the nurse responds. No one can get an IV setup that fast. We laugh some more. Real world meets theory.

I proceed to try to setup my laptop on the free network—some connection issues. Try a few things and no luck. Nurse hears of this and is having none of it. She dials up IT and tells them to get up here, now. She is great.

Tech guy comes up and helps me get squared away. I ask if there is enough bandwidth to stream Netflix and he says yes. He then tells me that if I bring an HDMI cable and have them reset the TV, I can play streaming movies to the big TV. Julie's ears perk up—"Michael would love that." I of course tell her to forget she ever heard that. Trouble brewing.

Pharmacist comes to explain all of my meds. Other than the four chemo meds I am going to be taking about ten other medicines.

Ridiculous amount of stuff blasting through my body. He is patient in explaining the medicines, side effects, and what all of the other medicines I will be taking will do to me. He super smart and patient.

Peed a few times in the am, flushed toilet and washed hands like a normal person. Told this to nurse and was promptly scolded—you MUST, MUST, MUST pee in the pee containers. They have to know liquids balance. He pulls out a sheet of paper that looks very serious and writes something down while shaking his head. I think I am in trouble.

Missed breakfast earlier so Julie gets me a breakfast sandwich and coffee from Au Bon Pain (no, I can't pronounce it). She tries to use her Buck ID card to get the discount, cashier scans it over and over but fails miserably as you actually have to have money on the card and use it to pay to get the discount. Lesson learned - $3.14 discount lost☺ but I win as the food was much needed and good. Everyone happy to see me eating. They are also very keenly interested in how much I poop. Great news.

Totally missed lunch—feeling hungry at about 2pm. Did get a very nice tablet to order dinner—Chicken Ceasar salad. The order process is great and the tablet has a ton of other information about my treatment, including blood chemistry. Too bad I skipped school the day they taught blood chemistry during my MBA.

At 3pm I get picked up by transport to take me to my echocardiogram. Girl taking me down is nice but speaks so low, you can hardly hear her. I later decide that the transport people are a bit sketchy. We traverse a lot of back hallways and several elevators and arrive at the echo place. Compared to the James, this place is not great, a bit more rundown but still clean and neat. As I wait I overhear a story from a guy who was burned in some farm accident, in a bed, with a wound vac and is insisting to leave—now, he says in the obligatory southern Ohio accent. Nurses talk him out of this very politely.

Echo guy comes to get me—not very good English but I can understand him. Cracks me up every time he calls out to get meds or other info and has to tell someone my name—"Boofman." In any case, it's an ultrasound of my heart. Never heard about the need for this test until this AM (more sandbagging), but one of the chemo drugs causes heart issues, so they do it.

Ultrasound guy is brutal. Ultrasound thingy is about six inches long and one inch in diameter. He put three leads on me, in the hairiest possible spots to remove maximum hair when they are removed. Then he applied the frozen ultrasound gel to the wand and starts the ultrasound of my heart. It was interesting at first when, without tears in my eyes, I could see the images on the screen. In short order, he started to press VERY hard on my chest to get a good image. Holy crap that hurt. He's done with initial screen and no ribs or sternum is broken yet. Now the funnier part. He calls to get an RN to help Mr. Boofman with some imaging agents that go through the IV. Step one, nurse hooks up two syringes to my IV. She sloshes something between the syringes to make the mixture bubbly, then wham—she shoots the whole bubbly mixture into the IV. Hurt some but at that exact point I am vaguely remembering all the bad things that can happen when you get air bubbles in your system. I don't die—this is good. Next they put some contrast gel in the IV—2ml. That was fine—but more chemicals in the body—you simply expel them through the lungs—allegedly. He took a lot of pictures and movies of my heart. I later find out all is OK. This is good.

Trip back to the room was interesting. Guy shows up after about ten minutes—at this point, I have to pee pretty bad. Guy taking me worked at a local company—in the warehouse. I ask if he liked it, he says yes—I ask, why did you leave. He says that he dropped an air drill on his foot and never told anyone. He finally asked to go home because of the pain, was fired that night for not reporting injury—all righty then. Next job he also loved was install tech at a cable company. Left there, allegedly, because the ex-girlfriend lost her car (I think if I asked for additional detail, I would still be in transit), and he was late to work after dropping her off so he was fired. We get to the James elevator and get in; we go up one floor (one nurse already in the elevator), and we stop at the next floor up on our way to 16. A gaggle of interns/residents following a doctor on rounds I guess waiting for elevator. They all jump in; we are crushed in the elevator. Doctor tells interns, "I think there is a 95% chance of no complications if we do the procedure." They all, of course, agree. From the doctor's demeanor, am guessing any questioning of that proclamation would be trouble. The lead resident is typing furiously on his tablet taking what must be very important notes. They only went up one floor, get out and off we go. We get to 16, and I get one final lesson on the finer points of driving a hospital bed from the transporter. Guy was great, easy to talk to, and got me to my room in one piece.

Get upstairs and the PICC ladies are there—super nice ladies. PICC is a long tube they put in starting at your mid bicep on the inside in a vein and fish it through your body to get to a main vein running by your sternum. If you are a doctor reading this—no commentary. In any case, they get setup. Take lots of measurements from my arm to my mid sternum then use an ultrasound (they are MUCH nicer with the ultrasound) to get sizing of the vein. Apparently I am a 27—which, as I understand it, is good.

Now very serious prep begins. They SCRUB everything nearby and get in full gowns. They put some triangle thing on my chest, right below my chin. I ask, of course, what this is. A "GPS" for the line— OK good explanation which I appreciate—got it. After lots of cleaning, they mark a spot on my arm with a tube and clean it like crazy people. Then some lidocaine to numb things, and away we go. On the monitor, we see the progress of the tube in my body. Julie knocks at door and is told, in no uncertain terms, to stay out—fainting risk I add☺ The "lollipop" on the screen represents the end of the tube which is in no mood to turn down the right path in my body. A few adjustments to my body position and we are all set and in place. They fiddle some more, tape it in place and I am done. They ask if I need anything—I am starving at this point and ask if they could round up some snacks. They come back with a pantry full of stuff—they were great. Turns out the "not hurting" is not as advertised—when the lidocaine wears off— the place where the PICC was installed really hurts. Upside is that the IV comes out now.

Now the main nurse practitioner comes in. I am thinking let's start the chemo, sister. She has some form that it looks like it was filled out and needs a patient signature—She says we need to talk. *Oh boy,* I think. She says I was talking with the doctor and noticed that you didn't get your bone marrow draw. This is the first I have heard of a bone marrow draw. Not pleased—more sandbagging. I argue against this. She argues for it some but admits we should probably talk to the doctor. I say great and get his cell number up on my phone before she stops me—wait, wait, wait, let's see if he is available. I, of course, have no compunction making the call. It turns out he is available (he is great about this but I would have called anyhow), and we place the call. He answers the phone from a "conference" in Orlando (I think it really was a conference). We talk for a while, and I roll over and agree to the marrow draw. Which, as I now find out, cannot be done tonight. I may be smarter than a fifth grader but probably not smarter than a T-cell cancer specialist. As I am on the phone, two other people barge in the room with a portable x-ray machine and take a chest x-ray to confirm placement of the PICC. Hilarious, they never said a word, jostled me around, positioned the machine, got the pic, and left.

Now, one day in the hospital, no chemo and an added bonus marrow draw tomorrow. Yay me.

Michael and Libby come to visit. Libby pilfers my Gatorade, gets set up on Netflix (watching *Friends*) and settles in. Michael, on the other hand is looking at all of the technology in the room. In extraordinarily short order, we impose a rule that he cannot touch anything that is red. Seems to work. He steals the computer from Libby and promptly pulls up some of *The Simpsons* funniest moments. The first was Homer lamenting that he had three kids and no money instead of no kids and three money. This is very funny to me. Julie hates the shows but snickers at that one. Next clip is where Homer is hooked up to a lie detector machine and a very serious lady is explaining how the test will go. She finally asks Homer if he understands—Homer confidently says yes, and the lie detector machine promptly explodes. Julie laughs hysterically about this. Is this a breakthrough with her?

Julie lets the cat out of the bag about the ability to hook up a HDMI cable to the TV in the room to Michael. Guessing no way I am getting out of that. Is nothing sacred?

Julie and the kids leave. Michael lobbies to stay, to no avail.

I am still awake so I pick up my medical reports to read the ones I have not seen yet. Learn a few new things about my recent visits but was proud to be noted as "pleasant and cooperative." My bursting pride for my good manners is short-lived, however, as some of the nurses that came by later indicated that these may be code words for the opposite. Am getting tired of reading, so I turn on the TV.

Captain Phillips is on FX. Navy SEALS jumped onto the scene—things not looking good for the pirates. I watch until I see "Stop the tow. Execute." Bad day for the pirates. Pirates dead—world saved.

Flip to next channel and *Hogan's Heroes* is on. Awesome. Col. Klink is in the clink for being a traitor. Hogan fakes out the SS and gets Klink reinstated as Commandant. Schultz, as usual, knows nothing. All is well at Gulag 13. This is funny stuff.

Turn on a podcast about toxins in your body. Probably have everything figured out now in case treatments don't work right. Safe to go to bed. Sleep through midnight, and then the next day starts.

TUESDAY—DAY 2 ROUND 1

I am sleeping—then I am not sleeping—the IV alarm goes off. Yes, it is loud. I call nurse, nurse comes in, turns on all the lights and resets the alarm. Great.

Now I am awake. I turn on TV and find CCTV4—Chinese TV complete with subtitles in Chinese (maybe another dialect or to teach illiterate Chinese?) and English. I wonder why I have Chinese TV. No clue. Really old guy is on teaching about health—so I start listening - I need health– he tells a story about a guy who moves from northern China to a warm weather place in southern China for the winter—this is bad he says because your body has to follow the seasons and you shouldn't sweat in winter—good advice. I am tired but amused and go back to bed.

I have good sleep until 7am—then breakfast came. Michael ordered it for me. I am guessing this is how an omelet morphed into a breakfast burrito. Tastes OK but not great.

Julie shows up with Starbucks—AWESOME. I drink coffee and get a shower. Ready for my bone marrow draw.

CNP shows up at 9:15 to start bone and marrow draw. Cleans up a bunch. Nerdy girl with a bucket of supplies shows up to do the marrow slides. She doesn't say a word but gives a curt nod not unlike a Lufthansa flight attendant—she is pathology. NP starts with cleaning my back (they take bone from right above your butt on either side of your spine). Lidocaine to numb me—that hurts. She starts poking— NO, not numb yet. More lidocaine, and off we go. She is grinding a hole in my back/bone and finally gets to the marrow. She pulls some out—it hurts but not bad and in a very strange way—kind of like a moving toothache. Anyhow, she then gets a bone core and that hurts some but feels REALLY weird. Feels like someone is banging on your body from the inside. Anyhow, she is quick, and I ask to see the goodies she just extracted. Marrow is gone as nerdy girl left right away. Bone looks like bone. Nothing special. Almost at same time I get done, Brad texts me to get the medicine to take the edge off before the procedure—good advice—late by about 20 minutes but good advice. Wasn't really optional for me—they gave me the medicine to take the edge off anyhow.

Nurse comes in with a small cup of pills, watches me take them—I am officially old. Ridiculous number of pills. I have them explain them all every day. I am not crazy—I want to know what is going in my body.

Nutritionist comes next—I asked to see her specially. I ask what I can or should eat to promote health of white blood cells after I leave– she is flummoxed—no restrictions, she says. This is a cancer hospital—right—they don't care what I eat when I leave. Sushi not great, wash veggies, no flowers, yada, yada, yada. Not pleased with this. She returns later with some articles printed from the internet and does her best to be helpful.

Chemo meds arrive and we get started at around11:30—uneventful. They simply hook it up and move out. No problems.

Julie visits again—this good.

Angela shows up. We talk for a while and she is lamenting her boy issues. Has not met anyone who is a keeper. I ask if she is on Tinder— she says yes but doesn't use it because she doesn't hook up. We plan an experiment to see who is out there. I, of course, will help her vet people. She logs in and has a bunch of people that have right swiped her over the last several months. One is 8 miles away—I ask how far away the local jail is—we laugh. In any case, the Tinder experiment is off and running. More news tomorrow.

Tom and Jeanne show up. Funny story. Jeanne asks Julie what room I am in. Julie tells her but also cautions of a long walk and that Tom should get a wheelchair. Jeanne asks Julie if she thinks there will be a wheelchair for him. Julie is confused—did someone just ask her if they had wheelchairs at a hospital? We all laugh hysterically. Glad we got that sorted out. Angela leaves.

Tom and Kristin show up. Tom has knee surgery tomorrow. We laugh about a series of things together and notice that the number of people from the hospital that stop in my room grows exponentially over the next few minutes. Since Tom shows up in uniform, I think they may have been looking for a juicy story. Nothing here. Sorry.

After some more small talk—things get serious. Kristin and I start sizing up the situation. Is it legal? Maybe. Is it advisable? Likely not. In whatever way we cite that no restrictions on diet should really mean no restrictions. Convinced, we forge ahead and we feel sneaky—that's kind of fun. Not sure we will opt in but at least we have a plan coming together. Gentleman Jack—does it even come in small bottles, or will it have to be rebottled somehow and "smuggled in?" This is to be decided. Cold Coke as a mixer is no problem whatsoever—merely a buzz away on the nurse call button—we agree this is an awesome development. A plan is taking shape—should we decide to forge ahead with a celebratory adult beverage. The term "outlaws" now seems fitting. Tom and Kristin leave.

Ortho resident arrives from my ortho doc's office to check on my surgical wound. Unlikely story as I am an anomaly to them, and they are simply curious. Lots of people "checking" on the wound now that the circus is only a few floors up. He makes the perfunctory check—all looks good (of course). Now engage in some idle chat. Undergrad Gonzaga, MBA Notre Dame (Julie and I immediately give each other the stink eye), IU for med school (at this point, we confirm that his parents are ridiculous for paying for his collegiate joyride—WTF), and finally OSU for internship. We ask, "Who are you cheering for in the Fiesta Bowl?" "Notre Dame," he chortles. Oh no—I nod "no" to Julie—let it go—let it go. Julie and I look at each other in amazement—ridiculous.

He asks if I am on the ortho rounds. I say I don't know and ask when they are. He says 5am—I say I am good, no thanks, and he checks in the computer—not on rounds but it's easy to add me. We start razzing him about cheering for Notre Dame—Bandwagoner and other terms are bandied about. In any case he leaves, still rooting for the domers. I am convinced he added me to the 5am rounds for the ortho guys— maybe we pushed a bit too hard on the domer fan. Verdict at 5am tomorrow.

Nice lady shows up a bit later with a new OSU woobie (go watch *Mr. Mom* if you don't know what a woobie is). Anyhow, she is a patient advocate and asks how everything is going and if I have any ideas for improvement—uh oh, totally the wrong question for a Six Sigma Black Belt who wasted a day of impatient time doing tests that could have been done long ago. She listens patiently to how I would rede- sign my previous testing process, how they wasted a day of bedtime at a "sold out" hospital—yada, yada yada—I unload for a good fifteen minutes, she looks tired so I stop. ☺ I am convinced she thinks I am crazy. I can't be too mad as she was the bearer of the woobie. She has no idea how I got on the woobie list, but it is a good thing she reassures me. She leaves.

The kids arrive. Woobie is on bed, and they all size it up. Once it is home, I will likely not see it again. Michael immediately locates the HDMI cable he sent earlier with Julie (she was advised, in no uncer- tain terms, to forget it but to no avail), and he climbs up on the ledge looking for the HDMI input on the TV. Whoa camel –I say - hold it, let's not do that quite yet. Ok. Michael—*Hey Dad, I brought something for you to play with. Oh, good*, I say—he pulls out some buckyballs— very strong, rare earth magnets. I look at the magnets then at the wall of advanced electronics charged with keeping my treatment in order. Not sure this is a great idea remembering something about magnets and electricity not always mixing so well. I recall recent experience when some buckyballs got stuck on the steel part of the waffle maker at home, we had smoke, sparks and a non-working waffle maker in short order. I confiscate the buckyballs and put them away. Next up, a trip to the bathroom for Michael—he sees a cover over the toilet— now off limits for everyone except for me to do my #2 business to limit chemo drug exposure. Anyhow, I explain it's not a big issue because I pee in containers and they measure it all day. He asked if it would help me if he peed in the container for me so I could get credit. Love that kid—extra pee credit in the hospital—epic. He will definitely invent something amazing someday because he really doesn't think like everyone else. BTW—no extra credit for extra pee.

It is great to see Libby and Jason. Jason is tired from practice. We all hang out for a while. Jason and Julie leave to chase the dogs. Libby and Michael discover movies on demand and stay a while—this is great. We put on some cartoon movie on very loud volume. They like the movie—I start falling asleep. They take off, and I go to sleep at about 9:30.

I check texts before I go to bed—Angela texts that we have some movement on Tinder—we can confab tomorrow. I am excited. BTW—Angela is my coffee buddy—I pay, she gets a peppermint mocha, and she buys me some Starbucks (I ask for something extra, extra hot) she schleps across from High Street and we have some good coffee each day—it's awesome. She lives in her sorority house, so it's not a horrible walk. Memo to OSU—get a Starbucks in the hospital—it would print money.

I turn lights out and curse the huge nurse computer screen with a white screen saver background that lights up the whole room—this place is amazing so one design miss is probably OK. PCA tells me to ask for another bed cover from housekeeping to fully cover screen and block out all light—winning!

WEDNESDAY—DAY 3 ROUND 1

Peeing like crazy all night—ridiculous amount (more on that later). That plus lots of visits to flush lines and check vitals means little lasting sleep. Nurses and PCAs are great—super people and always ask if I need anything. I feel a little bad telling someone who busted though eight years of schooling to be a doctor that I need a Coke…with ice but whatever.

Not added to 5am, rounds to with the ortho guys—guess the Notre Dame grad wasn't too mad—Go Bucks!

Breakfast comes at eight and smells funky—how can bacon and eggs smell that funky? Since they smell really funky—it's a no go I think. Will snack on some goodies and wait for my coffee buddy who shovels in at around 8:30 each day.

It's a big day for Angela my coffee buddy and me, we are reviewing Tinder matches. She comes in and we start sipping coffee. She hands me coffee with the standard name on the cup—"Best Uncle Ever"—likely getting this title because I am paying, but she schleps from fifteenth and high to bring me this coffee each day—and it's great.

We settle in and start the review process. To match on Tinder (as I understand it), both parties have to right swipe to "like each other," and then they can chat through the app. OK—got it, let's see what we have.

First up—a furniture repair technician from Grove City. It became readily apparent that this may be much more of a project than first anticipated. I really don't know where to start with this one and how did he even get right swiped. We sort out the details and decide he is a no.

Next up—a guy in a penguin suit—really. Am thinking of abandoning the whole project at this point. A penguin suit? Anyhow, I am intrigued as to how this could even be considered for a right swipe. He looked like he has a good sense of humor was the response. We decide no.

Next guy comes up—*I like your style; we should get married.* Negative Ghost rider. This is creepy and proves that looks—he looked OK to me too—can be deceiving.

Matt—803 miles away. Whoa, whoa, whoa. What the hell is going on here. How did this happen? Apparently you can swipe when you see someone local and when you move, it records where you are. OSU dropout maybe? Anyhow he states that his is getting ready to take a shower—yes, cleanliness is close to godliness but, NO—that's creepy.

The next guy has "super liked" Angela—not sure how this works. He lists occupation as an Engineer but he is only 21. I am not CSI or anything, but something smells a bit fishy. We review his pics—lots of Carhartt gear, pics with girls (BTW- Business Insider says this is a big NO NO and is sketchy at best) and a pic where he was WASTED, at least in my judgment. We decide he is some type of "alternative" engineer—not building bridges or rockets or anything like that. I think he is out.

The best story is for last—an athlete at OSU (name withheld for protection of the innocent). She kind of knows him so this is a non-typical "match." He has a lot going for him, but Angela thinks she may be able to do better. She is pretty and smart and super fun, so we agree the bar should be high. This opens a productive discussion. We review communications between the two, she recounts the experiment with her uncle, he makes some family small talk. This could be promising—nothing creepy or sketchy, and he is already, at least partially, vetted by a few mutual friends. We decide that he must have something on the ball, as a D1 athlete—he works hard, likely stays out of trouble, and has good fitness habits. We agree to evaluate additional communication and make more of a judgment call tomorrow.

Neal arrives, Angela leaves. She to send any urgent updates on the project by text—this is important stuff, after all.

Visit with Neal is great. Good to see him, we recount general goings on and talk about his soon to open business—Mammos Kitchen. Fresh, takeout, GOOD food meals for your family. Coming soon to Granville. It's fun to talk about this, he is a true entrepreneur at heart. It's a really cool concept. He has a lunch meeting at Hoffbrau Haus. *Mmmm, Beer,* I think. Immediately, the nausea sets in for real. I tell Neal no offense and buzz the nurse for nausea meds—she arrives in short order—take pill and feel good in about twenty minutes. That is surely a message from a higher power—no beer, at least for now. The plan with Kristin is now likely on hold. Neal leaves.

Oncology doc comes to visit—she is great. Super smart (naturally) and very patient. I ask a LOT of questions of everyone who I see, mostly to size them up—really not needed with the caliber of people here, but I do it anyhow. She sounds like the police lady from "Fargo" (the movie). She is from one of the Dakotas (da CO tas)—long "o" here. Then to MinnesOOOOta (Mayo Clinic) and then here. VERY qualified.

I tell her I am not a big fan of the PICC—it's basically a plastic tube with some small tubes on it that sticks OUT of your body—that's not right. I ask the Oncology doc, how can this be "optional." I recount how easily I can donate blood, with plenty of good places to do a blood draw, etc. She listens patiently. Explains that they don't like to take the PICCs out until ALL the chemo rounds are done. But there is an exception—hope springs to life—everything, I think, is negotiable. The crushing blow comes next—the only exception is for IV drug users. I am flexible but not that flexible. We get a good laugh, and she leaves.

Art and Matt arrive. Great to see these guys—loving having visitors. We have a good laugh, as always, and they stay for a while.

VIP patient advocate arrives. He was strong-armed into the visit by Andrea. He is super nice, but I am not his typical visit. He basically visits VIPs and make sure that all is well. He also worked as an advertising exec and in development for OSU—I get it now—fundraising. *No*, he says, *just checking in because Andrea said so*. He is super and stays for a while as I ask a million questions. Good to see him—will have to tell Andrea thanks for setting this up. Of course, all the nurses and PCAs take notice of his visit—this is good, I think, as they know exactly who he is. I AM SOMEBODY NOW. ☺ A VIP by association—thanks, Andrea!

Night meds, more stool softeners. Yea.

Guy comes by from Newman Catholic Center—offers communion—I decline, I'm good (would have probably have to take communion if Tom and Jeanne were here). Anyhow, I ask if he has any prayer cards—negative. Wasn't sure what to think about that. Anyhow, will take him up next time on the communion, I think.

Some other guy comes in—volunteer student who brings small personal things you need. I am good (already needing more storage for all the food and things people have sent). He asks how things are—I say OK—then I get his story (lower bar for him because he is not treating me ☺). Anyhow, he is a biology student, planning on med school and does work in a lab that lymphoma research. Now we are getting somewhere. The interrogation begins. I am looking for any edge at this point. After about five minutes of some of my best questioning of the day—I squeeze out the name of an experimental lymphoma drug—winning—then find out they are just starting tests on rats—losing. Great kid. He leaves, comes back about three minutes later and hands me a blindfold—we were talking about how light it is in the room, even at night from the screen on the nurse station. He recovers from the interrogation, shows back up and delivers the goods—he will make a great doctor someday.

Sleepy now—Michael is lobbying Julie HARD to come visit after dive practice—we think better of it. Sleepover is muttered for Friday—oh, boy. We will see on that one.

When I was weighed in earlier in the day—I found out I gained almost ten pounds in about three days. Maybe too small for the fat person room on Monday but not now. WTF? Not exactly eating three squares of Chipotle, ate a few cookies but really, ten pounds worth? Slowly putting two and two together. I feel REALLY full, and breathing is a little tougher. I hear "puffy" muttered from time to time. I look at the IV pump for regular (not chemo) fluids. Number is 100 and has been since Monday. I decide to look at the units. Its mL/hr. Ok, I start doing some math—this cannot be right. Pretty confident in my calculations off the cuff but consult Google anyhow. Twenty-four hours a day (it NEVER stops), 100 ml/hour is 2,400ml a day. I figure ml's are small but that's a lot of ml's. Long story short, it's almost five and a half pounds of fluid a day. I complain to the nurse who consults the doc and I get dialed back to fifty. Solid progress. Another negotiation with the chemo doc in the am—and I am down to 5 now—1/20th of the original amount. Gotta take some interest in your own care. Did the same thing with vitals—scheduled for midnight, got them moved to 2200 (military time reference here) so I could sleep a good eight hours (or at least try) from 10pm to 6am.

Thanks to all for all the prayers, support and visits—it means a lot, and I am grateful for all the good wishes. Hoping this gives at least some insight on what it's really like in here. Wouldn't go anywhere else at this point—amazing people here.

THURSDAY—DAY 4 ROUND 1

OK, I get it. Sometimes it's better to not come up short. It's kind of like landing an airplane. Short of the runway—big problem, on the runway, even a little past the start of the runway, and all is good. I can report that the hospital uses the "not short" approach with laxatives and stool softeners for cancer patients. Without putting too fine a point on the situation, suffice it to say that they did not undershoot in this area by any means. TOTALLY empty stomach now—thanks for that—maybe we dial things back some in this area. ☺ Am ready to start the day with a good breakfast though. WOW.

Coffee buddy Angela arrives, we hang out for a bit, but she has lots of schoolwork to attend to so we keep the visit short. We dial back the Tinder review in the interest of time. She has been studying, so not a lot to report there. It's always great to see her—highlight of my morning for sure.

Neal visits again—awesome. He looks dapper—has a business meeting nearby and comes to check in. We chat for a few minutes and he gets ready to take off. We are talking about working out some. He suggests a few burpees at some point, nurse (in room) is listening somewhat but becomes VERY interested at the mention of burpees. "Your knee hits the floor, its considered a fall so…that's a no," she says, "and falls are a lot of paperwork, so it's a big no." Hilarious—we all get a good laugh about that. She is great. Having visitors is really the best medicine. It helps the day go faster for sure.

Tom and Jeanne stop by again. It's a long trip and they schlep up to see me again. They have been awesome. I am hollering about the sizable pile of pills I have to take every day—they laugh at me. I am old now they tell me. I really don't like it. I have taken more prescription pills in the last week than the rest of my adult life. I go with the flow here but ask about the pile of pills everyday anyhow. Everyone pretty much knows the drill so they tell me what each pills does—again—as they check them.

Daily lunch buddy—Julie comes. It's awesome to see her, and I know she is running crazy. I always ask if the kids are helping at home, how is she sleeping, how are the dogs, etc. So far so good.

HUGE thanks to the people bringing food—that has been awesome for the family. Our kids eat almost as much as our dogs—the pool time stretches their stomachs or something.

She shows me a card from the team at Fisher (OSU Business School). Wow, great people. They all signed a "hang in there" type card with a gift certificate for a food delivery service– super generous. I read some of the comments—they are not the generic—"good luck" variety but really thoughtful and nice things to say. I would sweat for an hour to come up with some of the nice things they say. I haven't met a bunch of the Fisher folks she works with, but they couldn't be more supportive. Hoping to see them on Sunday.

I get the new chemo bag. Every time they change the chemo bag it's quite a production. The nurse gets suited up in a manner suitable for an expedition to the Fukushima reactor in Japan. It's a little alarming, after all they are pumping this stuff into my body. In any case, it's a positive milestone each day to get the next bag. One step closer to getting better.

The basic drill now is taking a shower after the new chemo bag because it's really the only time you can change your shirt. I don't want to take a shower and put on an objectionable smelling shirt again so I shower right after the new shirt. I really have no idea how you can get smelly by doing basically nothing all day but I do. They tell me it's weird smelling chemo sweat. Yuck.

In any case, I have to get pretty taped up to shower. Am showering and hear some non-doctor/nurse/PCA shoes walking around my room. Some shoes with hard heels, some visitor or admin type. Every nurse and most docs are in some type of Nike Air or other soft sole shoe. I am full of soap and decide to finish the shower then see what's up. It takes a while, navigating all the drying, etc.—even with the extra space allotted to the fat person bathroom.

I come out to find a note from Deborah. Bad news—I missed her again. Super awesome she stopped by, and I couldn't even be in my room—ridiculous on my part. Make sure you all tell her that I really am NOT here and paid someone 100 bucks to post my name on a room door. ☺ I will do it again in a few weeks to keep the ruse going.

Am on the afternoon walk and see my main doc. He is walking out of a room. He asks what my walking program is and we take off on a fifteen minute walk (it's a figure eight by the way). He asks a lot of questions—I ask a lot of questions (of course)—we exchange a lot of good information—he is good at that part.

He was at a conference with some other OSU docs presenting papers earlier in the week. I ask him how things went. He says—no lie—"The OSU team really kicked ass." This took me a while to process. I don't usually think of doctoring as a team sport or a competition, per se. But he and the team here does think in that manner. They want to be the best, as a team. It's super interesting to me and makes me feel like I am in good hands. He didn't say it in a boastful or arrogant way, merely proud.

We walk around the next corner and one of the PCA's dumps a cup of Coke with ice at my doc's feet. Not missing a beat, my doc reaches down and picks up the cup, its top, and starts looking for other ways to help. The PCA is mortified but it's no worry at all for my doc. High powered convention success juxtaposed with regular guy helping clean up a mess, not two minutes apart, define the type of people they have here. They want to win, be great, but they get that they are dealing with people and are down to earth.

Walk is over—so far so good on my treatment we decide.

Night nurse comes in with day nurse for the handoff. Here is your new nurse she jokes (male nurse). Everyone laughs. It's pretty funny. New nurse has lots of interesting stories about nursing school and how it operates. He was a PCA before doing nursing school, so he used that experience to figure out if nursing was a good fit for him. He tells me a few funny stories about smart, nerdy nursing students who freeze in clinicals because they can't talk with patients. Hardest thing for some people he says. I think back to the Monday student nurse and see what he means. His mom works two floors up and his fiancée two floors down. I meet the fiancé a little later and see a pic of his cool golden retriever. I remember when Julie and I were DINKS (90s reference—Google it). Fun times.

Jenny and Phil stop by—I appreciate the company, as it's a pretty good hike for them. We get caught up on the kids and talk about general goings on. It's rare I get to hang out with them alone, and I like it.

Libby rolls in from dive practice—dog-tired and sets up shop in my bed. Rearranges the pillows, grabs a woobie, and then finds some crackers and a granola bar. I FREAK out. NO crackers or crumbs in the bed! I have to sleep there. Seriously. She complies, sort of, by leaning over the bed while she eats the stuff with crumbs. Jenny and Phil leave. Great to see them.

Libby hangs for a while, a little too long for Julie (as evident by the calls and texts). I reluctantly kick her out after Big Bang Theory ends. She has a crazy schedule and needs to rest. Will be home soon I tell her. Long hug, and she takes off.

I start blogging. Then I get a VERY alarming text. Angela, coffee buddy, is "going out" with some friends to celebrate the fact that she finished her last final and papers. This spells trouble—I know it. Coffee buddy goes out late, and I am in VERY rough shape for the next day. I tell her have fun and be safe. Restless sleep ahead thinking about this. Very, very worried. ☺ We will see how it works out tomorrow AM.

FRIDAY—DAY 5 ROUND 1R

I am up early. Little sleep worrying about the coffee situation. ☺ I decide to take action, and ask for a Coke. I set off on a long walk. I surprise a lot of the nurses and PCAs walking around at 5am but it feels good. I tell them I am knocking on doors and running. They smile—kind of—not exactly sure if I am serious.

I get back, turn on TV. I scramble though the AM TV shows—they are all the same.

It's past regular coffee time. I fall back asleep. 9:30 comes, and there is a rumble at the door.

My coffee buddy arrives! She is tired. Really tired. But she came very strong and delivered the goods. It was great. The couch is pushed out some, I throw her a pillow and woobie and she lays down some. Peeking around the room—she asks if the can of Gatorade is spoken for—of course not—anything for my coffee buddy.

I'm not a big social media guy. I don't have Twitter, Snapchat, etc. As she is telling me how much fun she had last night, she tells me there is a Snapchat story. A collection of short videos strung together to tell your story. She pulls it up to show me. It was super funny. Nothing crazy—simply out having fun with buddies. We discuss how college students have done the same thing since college ever began (or at least since colleges were co-located with drinking establishments) BUT there was not any way to record the fun until now. It's a double-edged sword—I, of course, urge caution in social media. ☺ She laughs. She stays for a bit and has to go to work. Talk about coming STRONG after a long night—couldn't be more grateful.

Pile of pills come. They come on a huge ring every day, each medicine in individual pouches. It's a routine that the nurses deal with probably fifty times a day. We are going through the daily question and answer—what does this do? Is it optional? When the nurse find a problem—two pills in a bag of one. The pouches are apparently all prepared by robots—stupid robots, I think. Anyhow, I am constantly amazed at how careful the nurses are with the most routine and mundane things. She takes a pic of the offending pouch and gets everything straightened out. Somebody or somebody's stupid robot is in BIG trouble.

Nurse manager comes in with patient advocate. The patient advocate said she would bring her along to collect my feedback. Ok—but be ready. We start with some small talk and then get into it. She listens patiently to my suggestions. I ask a bunch more questions, and it's a good discussion. Conversation finally turns to the nurse workstation screen, on all night, with a bright white screensaver. Lights the room like a crime scene. What are the hospital's feeling about getting sleep I ask. ☺ She says there is a cheat sheet, somewhere, on how to turn it off. Cheat sheet? A long series of keystrokes are needed to turn off the screen. Really? She doesn't know how to do it but looks it up and makes sure my night nurse can (she comes back after we are done and checks it—as always, good follow up. I suggest an on/off button. ☺ Smart ankle comment—I know, but funny to all.

Things turn a bit sneaky now. She asks about the food. I say its ok and make some general suggestions, but it's really not her department. She asks me to report out on the nutrition people. Wants to know how that part of the stay has been and wants me to make observations, on purpose. A real spying assignment—that's cool! On the one hand, does she really want me to spy ,or is it simply a diversion so I stop asking all these questions of her nursing team? I decide to accept the assignment but will have to e-mail the results, as she does not work on the weekend.

I suggest Chipotle at least once per day for all patients. Some things are still not possible at this point. She says E coli. Got it.

It is late afternoon; I get a knock on the door from someone I don't know. "Some people want to stop in and give you a present." I am a little skeptical—did Kristin finally decide to forge ahead on the Gentleman Jack plan? No one called to say they were coming to visit. I agree, I suppose a present can't be bad. The lady said they would be right in.

Door barges open and a bunch of people in high spirits (I don't know any of them) ask how I am, tell me Merry Christmas and they have a present for me. Cool I think and go with the flow. Then they go out to a cart in the hall and bring in a new woobie!! Another woobie—I can't even believe how great this is. They had a relative that was a patient here, and they do this as a means of paying back. The woobie is really nice, gray cheetah print. This was surely a highlight. I probably won't see any of these woobies when I get home—they are hot commodities in the Boothman house.

Tom and Kristin come to visit. Great to see them again, they don't ever arrive empty handed, and their goodies have been a godsend—especially late at night. We hang for a while, and they take off to tend to their kids and dogs. It's an effort to come to visit, and I appreciate it.

Julie brings dinner—Au Bon Pain—real food again. It's awesome. She has to go to see Libby dive right over at the OSU pool, so it's a short stay. I will have a completely different food strategy for the next stay. Jeanne—get ready. I get videos of Libby's dives before Julie's phone dies.

Julie stops back after the meet—unplanned visit. We sort out the meet results—Libby is getting better and did well. The OSU divers took the top eight spots. The transition from gymnastics to diving is a lot harder than it looks—getting used to effectively landing on your head and being OK takes some practice. Anyhow, Boothman homestead is generally under control. Dogs OK, behaving mostly, kids fed and getting where they need to get, people sleeping over. Will be good to get back to that for sure.

Last blog for this go around. We will see if it makes sense for next time. Discharge papers in hand and waiting for IV medicine bags to finish—should be about 4P on Saturday. Thanks again to all for the well wishes.

ROUND 2 - DAY UNO (ADDING A LITTLE SPANISH LINGO TO SPICE THINGS UP)

Stupid helicopters. Lots of helicopters tonight. Pod D is actually CLOSER to the helipad and I am on the helipad side. I can actually see the pilots when they come into land. Anyhow, I start to notice the start difference in the helicopters. Some are loaded with a full paint job, a nice wax job, and are reasonably quiet (Lexus® helicopters in my mind) and some other helicopters are like an 85 Pontiac® Sunbird® with no muffler. Really, really loud. In my opinion, if you are in bad enough shape to need a helicopter ride, you probably shouldn't get in a helicopter that sounds like the Sunbird. In any case, these people are likely much worse off than I am so I think it's fine that they do what they need to do—loud or not. That said—it seems that a lot of people get hurt at night.

Blood draw is at 3am—all part of the strategy. Labels print at 0230 and lab processes first blood received first. I don't love getting this in the middle of the night but am not leaving the chemo start time to chance waiting on blood results. Blood draw—check.

NP and attending show up at 0900. They say I am good to go except they are waiting on the Epstein Barr (EB) test. This is important because while many people have the virus (latent), it can help cancer get started if it gets into the cellular processes. Let's move it sisters—I tell them. Call the lab. They got nada. I'm not starting at 1000—they have to talk with my main doc to see if they can start without it. Probably they say but need approval.

Attending doc stays for a while. I get her story—she is from a nice suburb of Chicago. She talks about high school activities and says she earned a varsity sports letter in, wait for it—badminton. I am speechless—and don't even know where to start with that. She throws in that her uncle is an Olympic badminton judge. I am out, no recovering from this turn of events—let's move on here.

Undergrad Northwestern—good, med school—U Chicago—good. Guessing she is smart. Fellowship at U Michigan—Ann Arbor. Julie is in room—stink eye immediately develops—I look at her and shake my head no—let it go. Now remember—Julie won't even stack yellow and blue plates, bowls, or mugs next to each other in our cabinets. Actually rearranges the dishes to avoid this—seriously. We let it go. Could have been a big diversion.

We talk some more—she is really great and, of course, super smart. Guessing that they have their choice of people at the James—they seem to pick well. Also found out that my day nurse was one of thirteen people hired after interviewing over 400. She says the EB test still isn't back but they will start anyhow—doc texted her to go. Risk is low because they tested for it before and it was negative.

Chemo arrives at 1200, and they hang it up. Off we go. Four days totally attached to the line now—at least I know the drill. When they give the chemo—two nurses verify literally every letter of your first and last name and every number of your patient number against the chemo bag. Along with every line of the drugs in the bag and the IV delivery instructions. It is poison, so they are careful. It strikes me that in the bag (about the size of a regular big IV bag—maybe a liter) there is only 0.9 ml of vincristine—probably ten drops—that must be super powerful stuff.

Eyes burn after about thirty min. I get eye drops– this didn't happen last time. Hoping there aren't a lot of these types of surprises this time.

Patient advocate arrives—I can't believe she actually showed up. She was warned. Seems like she genuinely wants to do good plus, she is smart because I am making her job easy—really easy.

I offer both problems and solutions.

We have some small talk and then get into it. Item one—green caps. On the chemo floor. They have these green caps that cover your port and IV line access points. They have a small alcohol sack that bursts when they put them on so they are both covered and disinfected—good combination. In any case, they don't have them in the lab where I get blood draws between hospital stays so they uncap my PICC line ports and then leave them uncovered. This is, in my opinion, not a fabulous approach and creeps me out. It doesn't make you feel safe. She takes notes—what an easy one here. We will see—I will have about a month with the lab guys to see if this actually changes.

Item two—The drug section of the discharge paper is an absolute dumpster fire. I actually said "dumpster fire" to her—she thought this was a little funny—or at least pretended to. I have a graduate degree and it literally took me forty minutes to sort mandatory and optional drugs. Which were OTC, already called in electronically or had to be prescribed by an actual piece of paper (scheduled narcotics). Wanting to follow the program is really hard with this layout, which I told her was likely designed by IT, because it was easy for them, and IT is always lazy. I really can't imagine some high school educated and really old sorting this out completely. She takes a lot of notes. Solution—tell some Black Belts to get some Edward Tufte books (Yale prof who taught a seminar I went to years back on how to present information—simply), and fix it. It's really hard to make things simple but this is really bad and at least a little dangerous I tell her.

Item three—Windsock on heliport is snagged on something and doesn't move or fill completely with the wind. She is confused, and stops writing. I tell her I am serious—I watched a pilot (with a Lexus helicopter no less) struggle to get down on the deck because the windsock wasn't sticking straight out in twenty-five mph winds (my windows were rattling) when they use that windsock to gauge local winds, especially with a lot of tall buildings around that redirect the wind—a lot. Complete confusion by the patient advocate at this point. Not her department? Not sure what I mean? I tell her write it down and at least tell somebody. She wrote something—not sure what. Poor pilots.

She leaves, and I tell her that I will help with the projects—and I mean it. I will suggest we work on the discharge papers in my next chemo round.

Jason comes to visit after practice. He is tired, but I haven't seen him in a few days. I don't like that. In any case, he is OK except for the pulled stomach muscle. He only did part of the practice because he got really sore. I am hoping for a quick recovery for him. He has improved a lot this season and deserves to get his shot in the upcoming meets.

I start looking for Payton Manning's cell number to get an HGH hookup for him now. OK—not really. For the record—I don't think Payton did it. I do think Cosby is guilty though. We visit for a while, and he takes off late.

I am totally jacked up—doing emails till midnight (thanks prednisone) and try to sleep at about 1AM. I finally go to sleep something after 2AM after learning about Oak Island—place in Nova Scotia where the British or some pirates buried some treasure—allegedly. I think it's real, but they never find anything great. Lots of chambers well below ground. Gold chain fragments. Stones with weird lettering on them. I hope those guys hit the jackpot—the world needs dreamers that kill it every once in a while—RIP Mel Fisher.

Stupid IV pump wakes me up. I was sleeping hard and am sweating. Slept a whole hour. They fix the pump, and I sleep on and off until about 8A.

Preview—Tomorrow is a great day. More on the Day Dos (Spanish lingo reminder) blog tomorrow.

Day Dos (Spanish lingo reminder)

I wake up sweaty, I smell funky—and not good funky. Chemo makes everything that comes out of your body smell funny, combine that with a depleted sense of smell at times, and you can really surprise yourself—not in a good way. I am ready for a shower but have to wait for the new chemo bag so I can change my shirt—practicalities.

I had a bad sleep and am in a bit of a foul mood. That plus the funky smell, and it's going to be a bad day it seems—wrong answer. I catch myself - you can't get in the downward spiral in your head—that's where the battle is won or lost. I see it in the eyes of some of the other people on the floor—wish I could help them somehow.

Door opens—Coffee Buddy is here. OMG! OMG! OMG! Unannounced and completely a surprise!! I am soooo happy! Talk about your day turning around in the span of a minute! It was great to see her—she has been hanging with us at home during Christmas but was heading back home for a bit and decided to stop. How great is this surprise? We hang out for a bit, and she takes off. Feeling better now.

Tom and Jeanne show up with a bunch of tortellini soup. I am almost 100% weaned off of hospital food at this point, except for breakfast (cereal, milk, fruit punch –yes, I am a kindergartner ☺). Hard to screw that up. The tortellini soup is a lifesaver—and is healthy stuff, spinach, tomatoes, and pasta. You can't beat that. We hang out for a while—ask if they can help tidy up the room—I say to leave it, it's fine—Julie will do it when she gets here. We laugh at that. I tell them I was serious—it's the first thing she does every time she comes to visit. Julie is great—I always have a clean room.

Julie shows up with more goodies and immediately sets to work—barking orders—moving things, cleaning, etc. All the rest of us laugh—the room organization binge is 100% predictable.

We hang out for a while and Julie takes off for the cafeteria to get some food. Dr Porcu (main doc shows up) it's about 6P. He asks how I am and how things are going. He is really a great doctor; I don't recommend T-cell lymphoma but if you have it—he is 100% your guy. He is dialed into to research (he knows the main person for T-cell lymphoma at the NIH, CEOs of a lot of genetics/therapy companies, etc.) Really great resources at his disposal.

We get into my case. Bone marrow is still a slightly open question. Results have been back but I haven't heard the whole story to date. They do three things to confirm you are 100% clear. Get some marrow, put them on a slide and see if there were abnormalities—no is that answer—I knew that about a week ago. Then they look at the cells at a more molecular level to see if there are abnormal cells in the marrow—there are (most people have some anyhow), but they found some so more digging. Finally, they look at the protein markers on the cells to see if the abnormal cells are all the same (clonal—bad) or different. In my case, the markers indicated that they were different. This means a general response to some body stress as opposed to a response to a specific condition (*i.e.*, cancer in the bone). This was really good news—after all that, he can call my marrow clear. Last possible big roadblock to a reasonably short treatment cycle is gone now! That's really good news.

He says we are sticking with three rounds of chemo then radiation—bad marrow would have been at least six chemo plus some other bone marrow goodies before radiation. Apparently you have radiation five times a week for a few weeks, based on some calculations of how much mass they want to radiate. He expects that where I have to get radiation should help me avoid sickness from it. Probably about two months from now I can try to get back to a 100% normal life. That's pretty good news.

Heard about the daughter of a friend of ours who had some complications from a tonsil removal—everyone send some prayers for Megan for a speedy recovery. Getting more convinced that the praying thing actually works. ☺ Let's send some love Megan's way today.

We eat some and celebrate some. The family takes off—then off to bed watching some TV. I expect to sleep better tonight for sure.

Day Tres (that's three for all you English speakers)

I have a decent sleep and wake up slowly. I schedule breakfast food at 8 every day, and I usually wake up at about 700 or 730. I turn on the TV—it doesn't work—I FREAK—the TV always works—never a problem—ever—two college football playoff games on today and no TV. I turn it off and then turn it on again—it works! Very relieved. That was going to be the highlight of my day. No way I can miss those games—kills a lot of time and is entertaining.

I am now officially Yoda. No hair. OK, maybe some hair but definitely Yoda hair. Only thing is, I'm not 900 years old like Yoda, and I'm not a Jedi, and I don't have a light saber, which makes it easier to pull off that type of hair. I tell Julie it's hot, and I get the fisheye in return. Amazing how fast it comes out. I got a haircut on Dec 23 and all was fine. About a week later—no hair. Never been bald before, it's cold and feels breezy. I WAS bald as a baby but I don't remember it. ☺

I choke down my daily pills and have some breakfast. I get a text from Neal—he is coming to visit. Total surprise. He shows up about fifteen minutes later and we hang out for a long while. Great to see him and get caught up. He takes off and gets to his day.

Art shows up to visit for a bit. We hang out some and talk about a bunch of stuff. Christmas, Bernie's Bagels closing, New Year's plans, and football. It has been great to see him. Day is rolling along. Really great day so far!

Julie shows up - two very important things in tow—Tommy's Pizza and Kefir. Gotta feed the beast. When we talked about lunch, I said that pizza actually sounded good. It's weird, some foods I normally love sound really good and others sound like they would make you sick. Not sure the dynamics in my head, but I figured it was worth a shot with the pizza. Good thing I did stick with the pizza—it was the most amazing thing I ate in the last week—soooo good. Couldn't eat too much, but wow, that was a winner for sure. Hospital food is awful.

We hung out for a while, and I decided to have some kefir. Kefir is essentially a probiotic drinkable yogurt that has twelve types of good bacteria (yogurt may have one or two types of good bacteria). Since they killed pretty much all the bacteria in my stomach with every antibiotic known to man, I decided to try to put back some of the good stuff that helps digestion.

Using probiotics is certainly not a point of consensus among the doctors and NPs. I received responses from "hell no" to "absolutely yes." I guess, in some ways, they spend their day worrying about killing bacteria, and here I am going to put some into my body, on purpose. That probably is a bit unnerving. It's not raw milk, people. Main doc says let it rip with the probiotics—I figure he is the smartest of the bunch anyhow, so I move ahead.

Amazing how much the kefir helps. I can feel things working again in my stomach. I will have more tomorrow.

I watch the games. Clemson is good I think. More choke by Oklahoma. This is a great diversion—eight hours of decent football. I turn on the Sparty-Alabama game. Watch for a bit, boring, I fall asleep. Wake up and turn it on again, only to see Sparty get monkey hammered. They look bad. Athletes matter—Saban and Urban know this. Five stars is better than three stars. Thinking this sets the Sparty program back a bit. Quite a blowout. Now the Big Ten stinks again. We had a chance as a conference and blew it. I sleep on that thought.

Day Quattro (4)—Last entry this cycle—out tomorrow.

I rise at the usual time. Get some food, and Julie calls—we planned to watch the Bucks game together today, we make some plans and she says she is bringing the boys—great news—miss the family a lot here. They all come down a lot, but it's not the same as being home. Good thing I only have one more cycle. Still can't believe it—so great.

I get discharge papers—basically they tell me get out when you are done. I am all set now. The main admin hurdle to leave is done. One more bag to hang and a short one after that and I am done. That short bag is funky though. It's refrigerated, and they give it to you really fast (30 min). It's a strange feeling, cold some, dizzy some. I had to sit for about 30 min after that bag last time, even though I was free to go. In any case—I am sorted with "the system," so I am good to go.

Julie and the boys are coming to watch the Bucks game. I am excited but a bit apprehensive. She is loud during games—really loud. Huge fan, football smart, and into each game. She has a history of unintentionally scaring children and dogs with loud cheering or jeering during games. I think each of our kids actually cried at some point because of the loud cheering when they were toddlers—hilarious. This will have to be managed.

The crew shows up with some goodies and we set down to watch the game. Nurse Michelle comes in and says she already put security on notice—she actually said it—we all laughed. Game starts and we are off.

1st OSU play from scrimmage is a nice pass play—Julie starts screaming—literally—the boys laugh hysterically and tell her to gear it back some. I remind her we are in a hospital. Lots of sick people trying to rest. *OK, OK*, she says.

Zeke gets the ball the next play—great run for ten yards or so. Julie jumps up and literally starts stomping on the floor in excitement—like a marching band member. I remind her that we are in a hospital. It could be a long game. We all have a short confab and agree that deaf clapping—waving hands in the air—is allowed for her for the rest of the game. She actually complies. We all get a huge laugh when we see her cheer now. ☺

We watch the game and they go to the cafeteria at halftime for some food. I get a Coke out of the deal. I take a drink, it tastes funny. Like I said, it's a crapshoot whether things you know you like actually taste good. I suspect that this contributes to weight loss. I can't explain the loss of taste—it seems as if some of the flavor profile is regular, some of the profile tastes weak and some is simply gone. No balance to the flavor. Another chemo benefit.

The game finishes and the crew leaves. Julie is tired. I know it's been a long week and, as always, people have been great helping out. The kids have been great as well. I am anxious to get back and contribute, at least a little, to running the homestead. Less than 24 hours now.

I put on the Iowa-Stanford game. I text Brad and tell him Iowa will lose by three touchdowns. At 38-3 now, it may even be more. Iowa is BAD—really bad. Night nurse comes in, she was here when I first came in. I know most of the nurses now—it's comforting, and they are all super nice and attentive and most importantly positive and funny when they can be. That part matters.

Expect a slow night, will watch more football—good time to be stuck in a room with a TV the last few days and have a good sleep. Last bag finishes at noon—then the short one, then home. 2/3 done with the inpatient part after tomorrow!

Thanks to all for your support and prayers. It's been really helpful. Constant reminders to keep pushing or that prayers or coming or that people are helping out at the home with food or whatever is amazing. We are truly blessed—thank you.

ROUND 3 DAY EIN (GERMAN LINGO THIS TIME ☺)

Up early, want to beat the rush. Yesterday was a holiday at the hospital, so I expect a bunch of people showing up today. We leave the house a little before 7 and stop at Starbucks. Need some caffeine.

315 South is a parking lot—accident plus rush hour. Should have left earlier. Worrying already. Car tells us its five degrees outside—ridiculous. Why the heck anyone would live in a place like Minnesota where its cold like this all the time in the winter is beyond me. We get to the hospital—loaded with electronics, clothes and food—it's almost like I am camping but I know what I want to eat and it's not hospital food.

Julie drops me off—line OUT THE DOOR at registration—#losing. Its 810, and I have a nine o'clock appointment with my regular doc. Plan was to get in registration early and at least get a bed secured. After sitting for about ten minutes—I get called back to register. Takes a few minutes, and I have to sign something. It's really a joke—they have a signature pad and tell me to sign. "What am I signing," I ask. "A consent to treat" they say. Could be voting for Trump or Clinton or anything else for that matter. I sign anyhow and ask the all-important question—do I have a room? Negative she says. I am on a really tight schedule due to an event for Jason on Saturday, and it's not starting well. I need to get started asap.

We trudge up to the fifth floor and tell them I am here. Get called back at 850—I am impressed—my doc is super busy, and I am in early. Nurses take vitals and tons of blood—five vials—not a record, but it's a lot of vials. While they start up all the procedures—I interrupt and tell them they need to get me a bed stat—I didn't really stay "stat," but it's a hospital so it sounds good. They are a bit bewildered but comply. "I will call right away." They finish up with me and send me over to the exam room.

Dr. Porcu - who is awesome—comes in toting some type of research assistant. Millennial type guy, beard, dressed well with nerdy glasses and a notebook. He is taking notes. We go through all the medicines I am on. I have only two left I have to take every day plus about ten (no kidding) optional ones along with some $87 dollar mouthwash to help with mouth sores. He asks how I am doing, how I feel, etc. Actually listens and sees if there are ways to tune my meds/treatment to make things better. Really like this guy plus he is smart—I (tried) to read his research—he is on it.

He asks if I have any questions—I pull out a list—literally. I have a few negotiation points in the list so I have to sprinkle the easy ones with items that MAY be contentious, so I start out treading lightly.

Q1—when do I get some hair—sprouts in six weeks, he says—not sure I believe this but OK—more hats, I guess. Don't like the bald head—hard to get temperature regulated in cold weather. Hair report later this week.

Q2—Can I get the PICC line out when I am done—he thinks some on this (apparently I ask questions kind of fast). I tell him it's creepy to have a purple pipe hanging out of my arm (he agrees), plus

I am getting sores from the dressing they put on it. He says OK but reminds me that they will have to poke me to get labs for the next two weeks—I am on board with this.

Q3—What is the radiation plan? He is not sure—he will refer me to a radiation doc. I ask him (actually said it) who is the smartest one—he laughs and even the nerdy guy taking notes laughs. At this point, I am sternly cautioned by Julie—"They are all smart," she says. Undaunted—I press. I don't care—I want the smart one. He rattles off a few names, and I put in my preference—we will see what happens there. In my mind—the smart ones are the ones who can wade through all the uncertainties of reports, labs, treatments, etc. and get me fixed up.

Q4—(easy one before the important one). Any restrictions on working out after this cycle is done—he asks what I am doing—triathlon I say—just kidding—merely machines at LA Fitness—he says no problemo. This is good. Not super realistic for next week because on days 7-10 I have to rest after going up the steps TO the walking track—no joke. It's crazy how weak you get with this treatment.

Q5—At this point he seems pretty agreeable, so I ask the big one. Can I get on a twenty-three hour chemo cycle instead of a twenty-four hour cycle? He ponders this some—(one of the nurses let it slip last time that this CAN be done). I tell him—honestly—if the efficacy is worse at all that I can do twenty-four hours—he thinks some and says it may be more severe (it IS more severe - but bearable—eyes water, nose runs, stomach feels less settled but otherwise OK) and says he can approve it. At this point (he already knows me—which is hilarious) he IMMEDIATELY logs in to the system to send my chemo orders and set up the twenty-three hour cycle. He proudly says—you are all signed off, so I won't be holding you back. He jokes some but is a super guy.

He asks if I am done with questions—we laugh some more—nerdy guy already has three pages (seriously) of notes and his hand is likely cramping. I am done—he has more things to tell me. Says they are FINALLY sending out my tissue samples this week. I ask about the process and ask if the tissue from the tumor is homogenous (the same composition across the whole tumor for all you non-Buckeye grads ☺). He actually says "good question"—I am proud of my good question—I make sure that nerdy guy captures the moment. He explains that you can't have any old yahoo from pathology get the samples—you need some PhD types to get the sampling right. In any case, my stuff goes out this week (allegedly) to the NIH and to two genetics companies for trials. I repeat what I understand about the two genetics companies do—he agrees I understand it. The thing about this guy is that he would answer questions for hours and not think a thing about it– really like him a lot. He leaves. Nerdy guy actually makes comment about how much good material he got, while shaking his writing hand—that's funny. Will copyright it next time and get paid. Julie and I are sitting in the room - not sure what happens next.

We flag down a PCA, and she says the nurse will come back. About a minute later nurse comes back—beaming. "We got you a room." Awesome! Still a ton of browbeating to get the drip started, but it's fine with me. They schedule a follow up appointment. May have to delay radiation because leg surgery not 100% healed. Julie can't even look at the surgery site—it's bad. In any case, he suggests Vaseline˚ to help it heal faster—I will have to check with the surgeon on that one. Libby was prepared to help me with the surgery site because, as she tells me, "I watch *Grey's Anatomy*, Dad." That's funny, but she is the least squeamish one in the family and was a huge help when that was needing attention.

We get on the elevator—doors open, I take a deep breath to get ready. I am ready to be done but I have four days on the stick to get done. It's a mental game, so I have to get right between the ears. One deep breath then go. Name on my door already—in super large font— larger than other patients—I think this is some type of code—problem patient or something—I think about asking about it but let it go. I may investigate later.

Nurse comes in—it's about 10:15—I tell her I am in a hurry—she laughs, but I persist, I am serious. I need to be out at 1400 on Saturday for Jason's event. I start with the questions. "Does the pharmacy have the chemo orders?" She checks and says yes. "When can I get the drip started?" She says the pharmacy says it will be ready at 1300. She knows what is coming next and calls them before I even ask to see if they can hurry up—no deal this time. Three hours of screwing around before I start. I have her confirm the twenty-three hour orders—these are set. I know the rate for twenty-four hours so if they are sandbagging—I will be on it. At this point she looks in the system to see my service team. There are two choices: Hematology 1 (Hem 1) or Hem 3. I will investigate and report what the heck happened to Hem 2—I think something is up here as well. ☺ She says—exasperated—nobody has you on their service rounds.

Seriously—I am on waivers upon ARRIVING at the hospital. Waivers—WTF? Waivers—defined for the non OSU grads - an NFL procedure by which a team makes a player contract or NFL rights available to all other teams. Basically, if a player is no good or a trouble-maker—they go on waivers. Hem 1 or Hem 3 didn't claim me—and I am on waivers. Awful. That plus the large font nametag—something is up for sure. Nurse assures me they can get me going on chemo without this because I saw my main doc in the AM.

PCAs come up and take vitals—had them only thirty minutes ago but they want their own set– I lost 1.2 pounds between floors five and sixteen—good start there. ☺ I may go up to twenty to see what I weigh there.

Nurse Manager stops and says hi—she knows I could be trouble so is nice to me I think. If the night nurse can't turn off the computer screen tonight—I will be sure to let her know. ☺ She is super nice and genuinely cares - I tell her with my nurse in the room that my nurse is great and is taking great care of me.

OK—whatever, I think on the waivers—I will sort that out later. I get a call from some number I don't know and don't answer—Julie leaves and goes to work. Then she doesn't and I hear her on speak-erphone coming back down the hall—my main doc calls her (after I don't answer) and tells her to get me on the phone (who even does that—he spent the time to track me down HIMSELF—love that guy). ALP? and AST? liver enzyme readings are off some. I need a liver and gall bladder ultrasound—GREAT I say. That's awesome –can I have two? He says I can start chemo but they want to do this. Whatever I say—up for anything at this point. It's really crazy though almost everything they do is to prevent something else that could be really bad. Every time I ask anyone but my main doc about the repeatability of some of these tests, I get blank stares. I have come to terms with the inherent unknowns in all of these tests and procedures—that's why I ask for the smart docs. ☺

My cell phone rings—it's the James main number. They call me to tell me my arrival time for the ultrasound is 545 tomorrow. I tell her whatever—they can come get me now if they want—she is confused—I tell her I am in room 1647 and they can send someone to get me now or at 545 tomorrow to do the ultrasound at 0600. How she didn't know I was admitted is beyond me. I tell the nurses to get the transportation squared away for tomorrow - I can't eat for eight hours before the ultrasound—she computes a midnight cutoff for food—I know clock math can be tricky, but I remind her that 2200 is the cutoff. She says OK.

On the stick with chemo at 13:15—this could work if I pick up about an hour a day for four days to get out at noon or so. Last bag (cold stuff) is thirty min plus getting PICC out is thirty min or so. Lots of cajoling to stay on schedule ahead.

NP comes in and says that Hem 3 claimed me off waivers. It was Becky—a NP I saw before. She shows up late in the day and is great as usual. Says they my records were jacked up because I came in in between cycles last time due to a fever and was effectively traded to Hem 1, even though I should be Hem 3. Hem 3 giving me another shot at being a patient with them. It's a one cycle deal, no cash up front but performance bonuses. ☺ Good to see a familiar face. I ask her about what the low liver enzymes mean—she seems entirely unconcerned. Ultrasound merely a precaution.

Jeanne and Tom show up with tortellini soup. Jeanne is Italian and it's always about the food. Can't go hungry—it's actually a godsend—I eat soup pretty much every meal now (except breakfast). It's pretty healthy and tastes good. Wasn't expecting the visit, so it was good to see them and get dinner delivered.

Julie stops by after work, and Libby and Michael stop down as well with some lasagna from the Nakasians and brownies. I swore I wouldn't eat any lasagna (really rich foods with a jacked up stomach is not great) but had several bites and couldn't stop—it was really, really good! Curtis shows up—looking sharp and stays for a while and talk about *The Big Short* and the "full retard" investing approach (buying any stock when the Fed is pouring liquidity into the market). It was great to see him—he has a life and didn't need to come, but I really appreciated him making the trip.

Night nurse is Kellie. She helped me before and is easy going. Never had a bad nurse here—even once. Will likely be up late due prednisone. More tomorrow.

DAY ZWEI (DAY 2 FOR ALL THE NON-GERMAN SPEAKERS)

Bad sleep—I get to bed at about 2:30am due to the prednisone which I got at about 1pm yesterday.

Nurse comes in at 530 for labs—I am ornery and really tired. Supposed to have ultrasound at 600, but no nurse can find out the plan from the ultrasound team—they should come to me I am told. I am not hopeful.

I am awake and can't sleep now. 800 comes—I am hungry. I am now coded "no food" due to pending ultrasound. Not happy.

Coffee buddy returns at 930—it's awesome to see her. I make the decision to be a bad patient and drink some coffee. Whatever. They missed their appointment time—not my problem. Since both the NP and attending doc actually laughed when I asked what the ultrasound would find—"nothing," they both said. "They do it to be safe." After those responses I figure a little coffee is OK. Probably costing me $5K anyhow. I don't have any medical training, but I do suspect that the poison they are giving me plus all the prescriptions would explain any liver issues. In any case, I have some coffee and hang out with my coffee buddy.

Ultrasound guy and girl come in at 1015. They are a pretty funny duo. Guy has been doing this for seventeen years and is pretty much to the point—calls me sir as he works over my belly with the ultrasound. The girl is about eighteen months into her job and kind of helps and learns some. Girls phone rings—somebody wants to borrow their cart. She discusses this with the guy doing my ultrasound—it's a nonstarter. Funny to see the interaction—apparently this happens pretty often, but she hasn't made it up the learning curve that you always start with no for these requests. Guy finishes the ultrasound—seventy-six images—some dynamic showing blood flow etc. I wipe off the gallon of ultrasound goo, and they wrap things up. I remind the girl as they leave that if anyone asks to borrow their cart- it's always a "no." The guy thinks this is funny, and they leave.

I find a PCA and get some cereal. I am starving. He hooks me up with cereal in record time and I eat it up. Get some of my carry-in soup warmed up and have lunch—right after "breakfast." Feeling better now.

Bag changes at 1215—the twenty-three hour schedule is working!! Good news.

Tom stops by after work—in his police uniform. I always love these visits—it's great to see him and hang out plus it always hilarious when he shows up in uniform. About five to ten minutes after arrival—a stream of nurses, PCA's and other hangers on stop by to "check in" on me. They hang around in the room a while to see what we are talking about, and I usually don't introduce him as my brother in law to add to their suspense. The brave ones come back after he leaves and ask if everything is OK. ☺ Funny.

Tom stays a while longer—we complain about the cold, and he asks me how I like being bald—I told him I don't, and my head gets cold. He says he has just the fix for me. He hands me a new super warm fuzzy hat with ear and neck flaps. Awesome police issue stuff. Super great present—I am loving it.

Julie shows up—good to see her, but I can tell she is tired. She gets me some food and stays a bit until an old college friend—Jeff—shows up. It was great to see him. Julie takes off and Jeff stays for a long while as we get caught up on what is going on with our lives. Good to hang out with people with really no distractions—really great to see him. He stays till about eight and gets home. Says he will be back before I pull out.

I am tired and ready to hit the rack. Go to sleep at about 1130 after they take the last set of vitals for the day. Am good to go till about 600 tomorrow, I figure.

Day Drei (Day 3 for the non-German speakers)

Stupid IV pump—starts beeping at 330. And yes, it wakes you from a dead sleep. I buzz the nurse and she comes in pretty quick to fix it. She also brings labs so I can sleep on though the AM. Labs take about ten min and I kind of sleep through it off and on. Nurses are always doing what they can to let you sleep—they actually get it and do their best to stay out of your room at night.

Knock on the door at 730. "Nutrition" brings my cereal. Sun is coming up anyhow, and my window faces due south so I start waking up. Pretty good sleep, IV pump notwithstanding.

Pile of pills arrive at about 9am—I know what they all are by now and am on board with taking what they give me. No more nurse interrogations—at least for now.

NP comes in and tells me my liver is OK (lab numbers are normal by now anyhow). "Did they find anything?" I ask. "You have some fat on your liver." "Is that a problem?" I ask. "No, everyone has some." Will have to work on that. Anyone know of the "thin your liver diet"? I think I need that. ☺

I suppose if they look at enough things, they will always find something. She starts pushing for the blood transfusion, my red blood cell counts are low, and they want to give me some blood to get them up. I am not enthused about this and elect to hold tight but tell them to bash me over the head if I am running into a real medical risk. They are concerned and pushing some but not too hard on this yet.

Coffee buddy shows up. So great—Angela is great company, and the coffee is a godsend. An oasis of good food in the hospital food desert. Plus, it is still one of the things that tastes good to me, plus the caffeine doesn't hurt either.

Jeff shows up with some soup. Really good stuff from a soup place nearby. It was great—I ate some type of gumbo—probably a little spicier than I should have but it was good. Stomach was not happy a few hours later but it was worth it. You have to eat stuff that tastes good while you can because it's pretty hit or miss on what actually still tastes good. Julie shows up a few minutes later, and we enjoy a relaxing lunch.

Diana shows up to visit. She has been great—helping with food and dog duty at the house. She tells me about how Piper (puppy) is doing, and I am glad to hear she is behaving. She stays for a while, and we sort out kid stuff and other goings on. She also brings cookies—which are really, really good. Great food day so far! It was great to see her—always great to have visitors.

Actually got a lot of work done today. Lots of calls—I never tell people where I am and keep things as normal as possible—feels good to get some things done. It's hard to sit for four days straight—not recommended.

At about 3pm, I start to get really tired. It's unusual with all the prednisone I get, so it feels as if something is up. Don't really want to eat either. Just not hungry. I expect that the red blood cell counts are falling and I may need some blood after all—I should find out tomorrow. I sleep some, Julie comes to visit but I am a bad conversation partner –half asleep. I rest for a while and get on a conference call for a while. Good call and felt pretty good after that. Watched some TV until 11PM vitals then go to bed.

DAY VIER (DAY 4 FOR THE NON-GERMAN SPEAKERS)

Slept pretty hard through the night. One of those sleeps where you are "out" and don't move at all. I am really tired when I get up and know that I will likely have to get blood now. Should get a better feel for sure on that count once labs are back.

Nutrition brings cereal at 730. I am sleeping. They leave the food for me. I sleep some more. Nurse, student nurse and PCA show up at about 830—suppose I should get up now—I am still pretty tired but get moving. Student nurses are pretty hit or miss around here. Most are really timid and simply stand in the corner—literally. But this one is personable and engaging. She also works well with the nurse.

They prepare the daily pile of pills—it's crazy—something like twelve pills. Some are optional, but I elect to take them anyhow because they help with keeping the bodily functions moving - you can sort out what that means. I also get potassium today. The pills are huge—they look ridiculous next to the rest of the itty bitty pills I take. I know the drill on the potassium - I had to have it last time for a few days, so I don't push back too much. Stupid big pills that potassium. Hoping they didn't grab some leftovers from the OSU Vet clinic.

I tell the nurse I will likely have to get some blood and to sort out whatever has to happen so I can get started with that. She looks at my blood band and figures that I need a new type and cross—they only last three days. Your type doesn't change but the antibodies in your blood do change some, so they get all of that sorted so they can get you the right blood products. I ask her what bad things can happen with the transfusion—she rattles off a few things that don't seem too alarming (shivers, back pain, headaches). Always better to ask the nurses these questions because they deal with it every day and will tell you things pretty honestly, unlike the docs and NPs who always tell you everything is no problem—nurses deal with the problems themselves so they know the real deal. She will have to call the NP to get the type/cross order squared away.

NP comes in. I know what's coming. I know I can be a bit difficult on optional treatments/medicines (no laughing from the people that already know this) and she knows this already, so we start off with some general conversation. I know she is setting me up for the push for a transfusion and she finally gives me the latest labs—RBC is down a bunch since yesterday—I can feel it. I am tired, and we agree that I need to get some blood. She was a bit surprised that I rolled over so easy on this but I told her—I don't want it but I am not going to be medically stupid about it either. She is relieved and gets things started for the transfusion. Signs me up for two units—I think she feels as if she has one shot at this, so she loads me up. She also gives me my walking papers for tomorrow. I like her—great attitude. If I have learned anything in all of this, it's that you have to be an advocate for yourself in here. There are so many things going on, and you have to actively question and manage the process from your side. If you have a family member who can't do that for themselves—be sure to step in. It matters a lot.

They hang the final chemo bag about 1000. Should be out by 1000 tomorrow! This part of the plan is working well.

Nurse, nursing student, and nursing professor arrive to do the new type/cross. I tell the nursing professor that the nursing student is one of the best I have seen and that she is doing great as far as I am concerned as a patient. Student gets a huge smile but I mean it. Some of the nursing students are downright ridiculous—they just stand there. Nursing professor tells me that the student is going to do the blood draw. Asks if it's OK. "No problem," I say.

Every process with your IV/chemo/blood lines is a huge undertaking. They usually pull out a big pile of supplies to get ready. Uncap line, pause pump, flush line, clean line, draw "junk" blood (mixed with saline), throw that out, clean cap, draw blood for labs, it's a huge number of steps for what seems to be the easiest thing. Plus, they have to hold so many different wipes, caps, syringes in their hands at the same time to get it done right—I am amazed when I watch it. It would take me an hour.

Student nurse struggles some but does a good job. Nurse professor is patient and a good teacher walking her through the procedure and what to do when things don't work out—my line was a bit clogged, so they had to flush it some and start over. Nursing professor is thrilled at this turn of events because it's a good "learning opportunity." Student is done and they put a new blood band on me. Should get results in a few hours and get some blood after that.

Have a shower—also a big undertaking. They have to wrap your line and you kind of hang your arm out of the shower when you are in there. It's good to get clean but not the most comfortable thing in the world. Will be so happy when I have the PICC line out (tomorrow) and can take a regular shower without worrying about getting the line wet. The PICC line is open to a main vein in your body so you have to be careful. You can't get any germs in there—big, big problems if you do.

I did promise a hair report—not exactly sure the logic on this as far as what stays and what goes—seems pretty random to me, but this is what I have experienced. Head is down to Yoda hair. Pretty much nada. Eyebrows—OK. Facial hair—gone—don't have to shave and wake up every day with a "close shave" already in place—that's kind of nice. Arm hair—still there. Leg hair—mostly gone. Chest and hair in other "personal" areas—mostly gone. Doc tells me things start growing back in about six weeks—we will see—I don't believe it. It's probably been one of the most alarming experiences to me—looking in the mirror and seeing a bald head staring back –even when you feel ok. Part of the program I suppose. I don't get too worked up about this, but I imagine its harder for women.

Nurse shows up with another vial to collect blood. This is unscheduled—they are checking for some type of virus. Never heard about this so I ask a million questions—"apparently" they check everybody for because it can be an issue when your immune system is low. Feels like a setup to me, but she seems unconcerned. Won't get results till tomorrow—when I leave. Not sure the logic there unless they send some other meds in to sort out those side effects if I have the virus. Turns out most people have a lot of viruses banging around in their body that really have no effect, until you get really sick. A little unsettling to find that out.

Attending comes in to see me. Asks a few general questions and then asks the wrong question—do I understand my discharge orders. Bad question. The discharge orders (which the NP already gave me) are a bit of a mess, especially with the medications. The medication list is simply an alphabetized list of everything you have on your plan—some are mandatory, some optional, some as needed and, in my case, some vitamins listed from an old OSU doc I saw years ago. He logs into the computer to fix things—but no deal—he is locked out because the discharge orders have been finalized. By now, I know what everything is and when to take it (or not). It took me a long time on the first set of papers to figure this out. Seems like something they should fix now. I blame IT—they simply do the data dump I suppose.

Blood shows up at about 1400. It's a big production, like the chemo. Two certified nurses literally check every letter of your first and last name and every digit of your patient number. Then they read the blood instructions to each other to confirm the bag matches the orders. They take vitals when you start and then the nurse stays in the room with you for twenty minutes and take vitals again. They are basically watching you and asking questions to make sure all is well for the first twenty minutes. This was uneventful. Once I am OK for twenty minutes, she leaves. She tells me that they rarely have any issues where they have to stop things. OK I say. Took the leap here on getting blood but would have had a really rough week next week without the extra bump here I think.

Julie shows up and tells me about her day—plus a good surprise— Libby is coming to visit. Daughters and fathers—that's a pretty cool thing I think. Anyhow, Libby calls about 15 minutes later to say that the windshield on the Pilot just got clobbered by a rock and has a crack in it. We sort out that it's not too big and it's safe to keep coming. Just one more thing to deal with. Julie is ALL OVER it and we have an appointment at Safelite* at 930 tomorrow to fix it. Good to knock these things out when you can.

Libby strolls in and comes to give a hug—so great to see her. She is super busy and I am glad she made the trip. We all hang out a bit, Libby takes off to her social schedule after a few hours, and I hang with Julie some. It's good to be alone with Julie but we are both pretty tired. We set plans for tomorrow AM, when I get out. I give a short list of food requirements to get ready and feel like a pain in the butt. Red Gatorade, warm—not cold. 7-UP, not Sprite, and it needs to be cold. Ensure—chocolate and vanilla—must be in the back of the fridge to get super cold. Honey Nut Cheerios*—two boxes. I know what works for the most part now so I want to be ready.

Lots of texts from people today checking in Nate, Anthony, Brian and Jeff to name a few - I am blessed. Always great to hear from people.

Blood finishes at about 2000. I feel much better way more energy. Hoping for a good sleep and an easy wrap up tomorrow AM. Should have the last creepy chemo bag (super cold given super-fast) at about 900. Then PICC line out and off a few weeks of recovery before radiation.

This is the end of the chemo blog since I am done tomorrow AM early with this last round. Hopefully it was a little interesting, a little funny and a little informative. If anyone reading this has to travel the same road (or has a family member who does), call me. I am happy to share my experiences with anyone to ease their apprehension. The battle is truly between the ears, and writing this helped me keep squared away on that count.

Thanks for all the well wishes—it has been amazing and helped more than you all know—thank you!

BONUS: SOME SOUP RECIPES AND ICE CREAM IDEAS

TORTILLA SOUP

I like it because it's not too rich, and you can modify the taste a lot with salt, cumin, chili powder, garlic, and Worcestershire sauce, depending on your ability to taste at the moment. Plus, you can add tortilla chips, cheese, and sour cream to the soup when you eat it. Good food and easy and clean protein.

Here we go:
1 Chopped Medium White Onion
3 Minced Garlic Cloves
2 Tbsp. Olive Oil

Chop the Onion and Garlic to the consistency you desire. I prefer to put the onion in a food processor and put the garlic through a garlic press.

Add the following to the Garlic, Onion, and Olive Oil:

2 Fresh Tomatoes (regular size—like a baseball) chopped to the consistency you desire

    OR

1 Can of Diced Tomatoes—15 Ounces.

Again you can leave the tomatoes as coarse or fine as you like. If you use fresh tomatoes, make sure you let the soup cook for at least an hour after all ingredients have been added.

5 Cups Chicken Broth
1 Tsp. Worcestershire Sauce
1 Tsp. Chili Powder
1 Tsp. Ground Cumin
Salt to taste

1 Lb. Chicken Breast—cooked in water, baked, grilled—whatever way you like. Again, cut as coarse or as fine as you prefer. Once cooked and chopped—add to the soup.

Let the soup cook for at least an hour.

Serve in soup cups or bowls and garnish with chopped Tortilla Chips, Mexican Cheese, or Sour Cream. Add hot sauce if you prefer.

Flavor Levers: Worcestershire Sauce, Cumin, Salt, Chili Powder, Garlic, and Hot Sauce (added if you like).

BEEF BARLEY SOUP

I like it because it has lots of good stuff in it, and you can load up on veggies (fresh and frozen) and modify the taste with salt or bullion by using bone broth (makes it taste richer) or fatty (or lean) beef.

Here we go:
1 lb. Lean ground beef
½ Large White onion, chopped or minced
2 Cloves Garlic, pressed or minced
2 Tbsp. Olive oil
5 Cups Water and 2 bouillon cubes OR 5 cups of beef broth OR 5 Cups Beef Bone Broth
1 Can Diced tomatoes—14.5 oz.
¾ Cup Quick Barley

½ Cup Sliced carrots
½ Cup Sliced celery
½ tsp. Dried basil
Salt to taste
1 Package of mixed vegetables—9 oz.

Use a soup pot. Add 2T of olive oil to the pot and brown the ground beef. Next, add the onions and garlic and cook until the onions are softened. Add all remaining items except for the frozen vegetables and bring soup to a boil (medium/high heat). Finally, add the frozen vegetables and cook for at least 10 minutes. Add salt to taste. Add more broth if the soup gets too thick.

TORTELLINI SOUP

I like it because it's an easy way to get lots of spinach and some tomatoes. You can add flavor with the type of tortellini or by adding Parmesan cheese to the top after you serve it. My Italian mother-in-law made this for me (it's her recipe) when I was in the hospital—it was really great.

Here we go:
3 Cloves Garlic—pressed or minced
2 Tbsp. Olive oil
4 Cups Chicken broth
1 Bag Cheese Tortellini (frozen or fresh)—10 oz. minimum
1 Package Chopped Frozen Spinach—10 oz.
1 Can Diced tomatoes—14.5 oz.
Salt to taste
Shredded Parmesan Cheese for topping.

In a soup pot on medium heat, heat garlic and olive oil for 2-3 minutes or until light brown. Add chicken broth and tortellini and bring to a boil. Reduce heat to simmer and add spinach and tomatoes and cook for another 10 minutes. Add salt to taste. When serving, add parmesan as a topping.

CHOCOLATE CHIP COOKIES

I like them because the contain chocolate and lots of fiber via the oats—when you are ready for it. You can tweak the flavor some with more vanilla, more sugar, more chocolate chips, or more salt, depending on your tastes. Try some dough before you bake to take a crack at what taste may be missing for you.

Here we go (make a half recipe if you must):
2 Cups Butter
4 Cups Flour
2 Tsp. Baking Soda
2 Cups Sugar
5 Cups Blended Oatmeal (put oatmeal in a blender until it is the consistency of flour)
24 Oz. Chocolate Chips (spend the extra buck and get Ghirardelli or Nestle)
2 Cups Brown Sugar
1 Tsp. Salt
4 Eggs
2 Tsp. Baking Powder
2 Tsp. Vanilla Extract (real extract—not the fake stuff)

Flavor levers: more salt, more vanilla, more sugar, or more chips.

Blend the Oatmeal in a blender to a fine powder—set aside

Cream Butter and both sugars

Add Eggs, Vanilla and mix together with Flour, Oatmeal, Salt, Baking Powder, and Baking Soda. Add in Chocolate Chips.

Make dough balls for cookies. (Taste the dough and adjust ingredients some if needed).

Bake at 375 Degrees for 10 minutes. Makes 100+ cookies.

ICE CREAM IDEAS

Living in Powell, Ohio, is awesome from an ice cream point of view. We have three world-class ice cream stores in our town, and all of the companies are based in Ohio. There are a bunch of other custard and ice cream operations in Powell as well. It's the best.

Ordering ice cream from far away is expensive; I get it. Do it anyway if you can. Here are my suggestions.

HANDEL'S

My "go-to" ice cream was Handel's. Very creamy and lots of good flavors. For some reason, this seemed creamier to me when I was craving ice cream, and it helped me taste the flavors better (I know, not very scientific, but that's what I felt).

Order here: https://handelsicecream.com

MY OTHER TWO FAVORITES: GREATER'S AND JENI'S

In my opinion, Greater's has the best "chip" ice creams—the chips aren't a uniform size, so you may get some huge chunks instead. Raspberry chip is the best. Order here: https://www.graeters.com

Jeni's is the hometown ice cream (Columbus, Ohio). Given that your taste buds are a bit strange during treatment, I always stayed in the fairway with their flavors (you will understand this if you order some ice cream from them). Buckeye State and Salty Caramel are my favorites. Order here: https://jenis.com

LIQUID NITROGEN ICE CREAM

Dear Science Nerds or Friends of Science Nerds—if you know someone who can get their hands on a liquid nitrogen dewar—have them get it filled and make some liquid nitrogen ice cream for you. It's the absolute best—but you have to eat it fresh. I have a dewar and made the ice cream all the time when my kids were younger.

IMPORTANT: If you don't know what you are doing with liquid nitrogen, then don't do it. It's a little dangerous so sort out how to be safe with it from someone who knows how to handle it.

Here we go:
2 Cups Milk (whole or 2%)
3 Cups Heavy Cream
½ Cup Sugar
2 Tbsp Vanilla Extract

For Chocolate Ice Cream add:
½ Cup Cocoa Powder
¼ Cup Sugar (additional)

We used the KitchenAid® mixer with the stainless steel bowl to mix this.

Put everything in the mixer bowl and slowly add the liquid nitrogen (so it doesn't splash) to the mixture until the ice cream gets to the desired consistency. USE GLOVES to handle the bowl when serving.

It's expensive but is very quick to make and tastes really great.

One last thought—a few good cookbooks were recommended to me:

1. *Eating Well Through Cancer: Easy Recipes and Recommendations During and After Treatment* by Holly Clegg and Gerald Miletello
2. *Chemo Kitchen* by Cal McAllister

ABOUT THE AUTHOR

Being highly observant is both a blessing and a curse.

—Jeff Boothman

I have spent the better part of my adult life in leadership and operations roles at companies, both big and small. What does that mean exactly? It means I have led teams of people responsible for you being able to get a light bulb at Walmart, gas at service stations in Boston, oil to your refinery in California, packaging material to ship your breakable items, industrial diamonds to make your granite counter, and your new professional-grade toolbox, among other things. It also means I have been programmed, for years, to notice details that are out of place.

Making these everyday occurrences happen is not always pretty; it's usually hard work with a LOT of attention to often mundane details constantly managed by very dedicated people.

If you move into one of these roles for the first time, you either live or die (functionally) very quickly. It requires you to recognize, synthesize, and judge a large amount of material and detail very rapidly and make decisions, usually lots of them. After being battle-hardened in these roles, you notice typos, dates that slip, lot sizes that change, lead times that slip, delivery dates that show up as being on a Sunday or holiday, and everything else that seems "off."

In my case, when my wife tells me I can't turn it off, she is right. What she means is that I am always noticing things that are new to me, out of place, used incorrectly, or novel. You can imagine how that worked as I traveled through my cancer journey—everything was new, and there were a LOT of things to notice. Those types of observations form the basis for this book.

Here's how this type of constant attention to detail helps me spot things that are "out of place" as I go through my everyday life:

- A local restaurant posts how much time people can spend at the table for parties of six or more and parties of less than five. This doesn't add up for me because what if you have a party of five, like my family?
- Someone is looking for contractor recommendation because they want to redo "there" kitchen—oops.
- A newscaster says that 300 million children under twelve live in poverty in the US. To me, this seems like an awfully large proportion of kids in the country. In 2020, the US population was about 330 million. That would mean that not only is 90% of the TOTAL US population under twelve but they all live in poverty, which is unlikely.

And so it goes. Later in this book, I will recount a calculated remark by one of my docs about "medicine" treating my tumor—it turns out it was a sign of big trouble ahead. The mindset that constantly parses detail and checks and double-checks assumptions is truly a blessing and a curse.

It turns out I couldn't switch off my constant stream of observations during my cancer journey either. That's how we got here—that and some blogging.

As you move into leadership roles, your focus shifts more to coaching, training, people development, and strategy. My cancer experience, the goal to leverage my learnings and the desire to give back are where this book came from.

For those who are interested, I have one awesome wife, three great kids, and two really active Labrador Retrievers. I live near Columbus, Ohio, on seven acres (working to turn it into a farm). I earned undergraduate degrees in Finance and Accounting, an MBA in Operations, and I am a certified Six Sigma Black Belt.

See more at jeffboothman.com.

Do you have ideas on how to make this book even better?

Let us know by reaching out via email!
Ideas@jeffboothman.com

Printed in Great Britain
by Amazon

58946429R00098